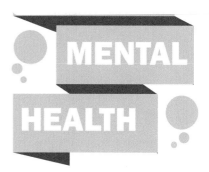

STAYING MENTALLY HEALTHY DURING YOUR TEACHING CAREER

POSITIVE MENTAL HEALTH

This series of texts presents a modern and comprehensive set of evidence-based strategies for promoting positive mental health in educational settings. There is a growing prevalence of mental ill-health among the teaching profession within a context of funding cuts, strained services, constant change and an increasing workload. The series recognises the complexity of the issues involved, the vital role that teachers and leaders play, and the current education and health policy frameworks in order to provide practical guidance fully under-pinned by the latest research.

You might also like:

Positive Mental Health for School Leaders by Jonathan Glazzard and Samuel Stones, Critical Publishing, 2020, ISBN: 978-1-913063-01-6

Our titles are also available in a range of electronic formats. To order, or for details of our bulk discounts, please go to our website www. criticalpublishing.com or contact our distributor, NBN International, 10 Thornbury Road, Plymouth PL6 7PP, telephone 01752 202301 or email orders@nbninternational.com.

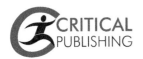

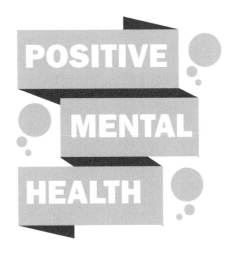

POSITIVE MENTAL HEALTH

STAYING MENTALLY HEALTHY DURING YOUR TEACHING CAREER

Samuel Stones and Jonathan Glazzard

First published in 2020 by Critical Publishing Ltd

British Library Cataloguing in Publication Data
A CIP record for this book is available from the British Library

ISBN: 978-1-913063-05-4

This book is also available in the following e-book formats:

MOBI ISBN: 978-1-913063-06-1
EPUB ISBN: 978-1-913063-07-8
Adobe e-book ISBN: 978-1-913063-08-5

Cover and text design by Out of House Limited
Project Management by Newgen Publishing UK
Print managed and manufactured by Jellyfish Solutions

Critical Publishing
3 Connaught Road
St Albans
AL3 5RX

www.criticalpublishing.com

Paper from responsible sources

+ CONTENTS

MEET THE SERIES EDITOR AND AUTHORS PAGE VII

INTRODUCTION PAGE 01

+MEET THE SERIES EDITOR AND AUTHORS

JONATHAN GLAZZARD

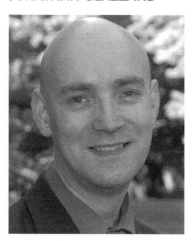

Jonathan Glazzard is Professor of Inclusive Education at Leeds Beckett University. He is series editor for the Positive Mental Health series by Critical Publishing. Jonathan's research explores issues of inclusion, exclusion, marginalisation, disability, sexuality and mental health for children and young people. He is a researcher, teacher, educator and author. Jonathan's background is in primary teaching and he is a Trustee on several multi-academy trusts.

SAMUEL STONES

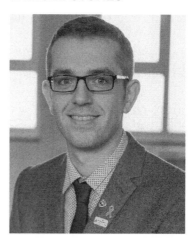

Samuel Stones is a lecturer, researcher and doctoral scholarship student at Leeds Beckett University. He has co-authored texts for several publishers and has written extensively on inclusion and mental health. Samuel's research explores issues of inclusion, exclusion, marginalisation, sexuality and mental health for children and young people. He is a senior examiner and experienced assessor and also holds a national training role with a large multi-academy trust.

✚ INTRODUCTION

The problem of teacher stress is not unique to England. It can result in teachers experiencing exhaustion, burnout and poor mental health and it can lead to teacher attrition.

This book provides comprehensive and practical advice to teachers at all stages of their careers to support them to be mentally healthy. It examines a variety of themes, including managing workload and relationships, resilience, time management, work–life balance and applying for teaching posts. Teachers can take control of some of the factors that can lead to poor mental health. However, some of the contributing factors require a systemic approach that addresses aspects of the wider education system and school cultures which have a detrimental impact on teachers' mental health.

Globally, teachers are currently working within a challenging education climate in which they are expected to compensate for societal problems and raise educational attainment, irrespective of students' backgrounds and other circumstances which may account for low educational attainment. Although this policy climate is admirable and promotes equality and social justice, it places significant pressure on teachers to counteract the effects of adverse childhood experiences and social deprivation. This can be challenging for teachers who work in schools that have high levels of social and cultural diversity. For teachers who work in affluent contexts, significant pressure from parents and school leaders to raise educational attainment can contribute to high levels of stress. The issues vary from school to school but the effect on teachers is remarkably similar irrespective of their different school contexts. Research demonstrates that teachers with poor mental health experience stress, anxiety, depression, insomnia, panic attacks, poor work–life balance and relationship difficulties.

Poor mental health in teachers is not a sign of weakness. It is an indication that something needs to change within the education system and within schools so that they are able to thrive. The costs of poor teacher mental health are devastating to the individuals, their families, their students and their schools. School leaders therefore have a responsibility to create positive school cultures which enable teachers

1

to thrive. This book argues that high teacher workload is only part of the problem. Teachers thrive when they are assigned agency, when they are trusted to do their jobs, when their strengths are recognised and valued and when they work within school environments which promote collegiality and openness. School culture is therefore a significant factor that influences teacher mental health.

The fact that roughly a third of teachers in England who qualify leave the profession within the first five years is deeply concerning, not only to the individuals concerned but also to their schools, students and society. High rates of teacher attrition are not universal and policy makers need to examine what is happening elsewhere to support teachers to thrive and keep them in the profession. In England, education policy in recent years has resulted in a gradual deprofessionalisation and general distrust of teachers. This has restricted teacher agency and contributed to poor teacher mental health and poor teacher retention. Teachers have been subjected to heightened levels of accountability and external scrutiny through school inspections, standardised testing, the national curriculum and performance-related pay. The marketisation of education has fostered a climate of competition between schools and consequently educational 'outputs' have been given greater emphasis than the process of learning. The new Ofsted inspection framework offers some hope that some of these issues can be addressed with its greater focus on the quality of education rather than quantitative measures of student achievement. We can only wait and see as to how this plays out over the next few years.

This book provides you with a 'warts and all' picture of teaching. It does not shy away from identifying the issues that you will experience. Nevertheless, it offers strategies for addressing these so that you can take control of your own mental health.

Samuel Stones and Jonathan Glazzard

✚ CHAPTER 1
CONTEXT

PROFESSIONAL LINKS

This chapter addresses the following:

In 2018, the Education Support Partnership (ESP) published the *Teacher Wellbeing Index 2018*. This chapter presents some of the data from this report.

CHAPTER OBJECTIVES

By the end of this chapter you will understand:

+ the extent of mental ill-health in teachers;

+ the factors which result in mental ill-health in teachers.

INTRODUCTION

This chapter outlines some of the factors that result in mental ill-health in teachers. You will also learn about the factors that can protect you from developing mental ill-health. Teaching is an extremely rewarding yet challenging profession. During your teaching career it is inevitable that you will experience stress. Teaching is demanding, and there will be times when the workload feels overwhelming. Not all stress is bad for you. Sometimes, stress can be motivating; it enables you to achieve your goals and complete tasks. However, when stress becomes overwhelming, it can prevent you from functioning normally and this can have a detrimental effect on your mental health. As a result of your work as a teacher, you may also experience anxiety, depression and other forms of mental ill-health. Unreasonable workload is a significant factor which affects teachers' mental health. However, this chapter also introduces you to other factors which are more significant than workload.

In England, too many early career teachers leave teaching within five years of qualifying (ESP, 2018). This is a significant waste of public and private investment and a loss of potential. Many teachers do not want to leave the profession. They leave because they feel that they have no other choice. While it is laudable that the government is taking steps to improve children and young people's mental health, more needs to be done to ensure that teachers are mentally healthy. Mentally healthy teachers are able to thrive in the classroom; they are in a stronger position to teach well and to ensure that their students make progress. Mentally healthy teachers are also well placed to support mental ill-health in children and young people. Teachers with mental ill-health can still teach well and their students can thrive but they are at increased risk of burnout and poor health.

This chapter addresses the extent of teacher mental ill-health and key themes which can affect teachers' mental health, including school culture, agency and workload.

THE EXTENT OF TEACHER MENTAL ILL-HEALTH

In the recent *Teacher Wellbeing Index* by the Education Support Partnership (2018), education professionals were found to be most dissatisfied with the workload associated with their job roles, closely followed by unnecessary paperwork and poor student behaviour. The data indicate that over a third of education professionals felt stressed with their jobs; 56 per cent experienced insomnia, 51 per cent experienced depression and 50 per cent experienced anxiety. Staff with up to five years' service reported the most mental health issues and senior leaders reported that they had experienced behavioural, physical and psychological symptoms because of their work.

SCHOOL CULTURE

The school culture is critical to the well-being of everyone who is a member of the school community. A positive school culture should enable everyone who belongs to that community to thrive. School culture is multifaceted but engendering a sense of belonging is critical to promoting positive well-being. The school leadership team is responsible for establishing the school culture and monitoring the extent to which the school values are borne out in practice. If you feel that you belong to a school, that you are valued, respected and have a right to be there, then you are more likely to thrive in your role. If you experience a sense of inclusion, this will impact positively on your well-being. In schools where positive cultures exist, teachers feel appreciated, are trusted to carry out their duties and are treated as professionals; they are empowered to further develop as teachers and will demonstrate high levels of commitment.

A climate of openness is critical to a positive school culture. You should feel able to talk about your own mental health without feeling that you are being judged negatively by others. You should be able to talk to other colleagues about the professional or personal challenges that you are experiencing without feeling that your disclosures will result in negative appraisal of your work as a teacher. Within positive school cultures, colleagues work collaboratively to support each other through personal and professional challenges. This includes providing support to colleagues for the management of student behaviour. Within positive school cultures, judgement is suspended and staff work collegially to offer mutual support, advice and development.

If staff are treated like adults, rather than as children, they will not feel patronised and will be more motivated in their roles. Within positive school cultures, individuals are not blamed for things that go wrong. Instead, there is a sense of collective responsibility in which everyone works collegially for the greater good of the staff team, the students and the school. Gossip and 'back-stabbing' are rooted out and challenged to prevent the development of a corrosive, toxic culture which undermines people's confidence, self-worth and well-being.

Teacher resilience is not only influenced by school climate. Research demonstrates that teachers are more resilient to the demands of the job when they have a sense of mortal purpose and vocation (Beltman et al, 2011). Thus, teachers who are exposed to negative school climates can survive and thrive if they have a deep commitment to the profession and to their students.

CRITICAL QUESTIONS

+ What other factors contribute to the development of a positive school culture?
+ What factors might cause a school culture to change from a positive to a negative culture?
+ How might negative school cultures affect staff well-being?
+ How might negative school cultures affect learning and teaching?
+ Reflect on your own school context. How would you describe the school culture and what factors contribute to this?

TEACHER AGENCY

Teachers have agency when they feel in control of their job role and when they are able to actively shape that role. Thus, when teachers are not able to make decisions about how to teach, their agency becomes restricted and this results in their deprofessionalisation. Lack of professional autonomy can result in teacher burnout (Skaalvik and Skaalvik, 2009).

Schools are complex social systems which impose structures on teachers. School policies shape pedagogical approaches and therefore limit teacher agency. In addition, the national curriculum is also structural; it specifies the curricular content that teachers are legally required to teach and this, in turn, influences pedagogy in classrooms. Also, national and local assessment policies specify national standards and approaches to assessment that teachers are required to adopt. These also limit teacher agency.

As a teacher you operate within tightly defined structures but there is still space for giving teachers agency. Your agency is severely restricted when there is unnecessary over-prescription on how to plan lessons and how to sequence learning and structure lessons and when you are instructed to use specific pedagogical approaches. While the national curriculum specifies the content that must be taught and national assessment benchmarks specify the standards which must be achieved, you should be given opportunities to make your own decisions about how to structure content, which pedagogical approaches to use in the classroom and how to monitor students' progress towards the national standards. Removing these decisions from you can result in demotivation, loss of self-worth and poor well-being.

CRITICAL QUESTIONS

+ Is it ever appropriate to restrict teacher agency? Explain your answer.

+ How might teacher agency change throughout your career as a teacher?

+ How much agency do teachers have in your own school and what factors contribute to this?

TRUST

When teachers feel trusted to do their jobs, they are likely to be more motivated, more productive and have a positive sense of well-being. Lack of trust results in teachers being micro-managed and this limits teacher agency.

CRITICAL QUESTIONS

+ What factors might make it difficult for senior leaders to trust teachers?

+ What factors might result in loss of trust towards a teacher?

+ What factors might result in greater trust being assigned to a teacher?

+ How can senior leaders gain the trust of their staff?

+ How much trust do senior leaders assign to staff in your own school context and what factors influence this?

ACCOUNTABILITY

As a teacher you are accountable to a range of stakeholders for the quality of your teaching and the progress and attainment of your students. Stakeholders include your line manager, the leadership team, school governors, the local authority or multi-academy trust, parents and students. In recent years, the level of accountability on teachers has increased and excessive accountability can cause teachers to develop mental ill-health. The pressures on you as a teacher to accelerate student progress and drive up attainment will be significant. Constant learning walks, lesson observations and monitoring of work in students' books can result in mental ill-health in teachers, especially if these are not conducted fairly and if you are made to feel inadequate. You will be required to explain the progress data of your students at least a minimum of once every term. Although a range of factors can influence students' progress, many of which may be outside of the control of teachers, some teachers may be blamed for lack of progress and this can affect their own well-being.

CRITICAL QUESTIONS

+ What do you think constitutes 'reasonable' accountability for teachers?

+ What factors have led to teacher accountability increasing over the past three decades?

+ What accountability mechanisms exist in your school and are these reasonable?

TEACHER WORKLOAD

Teaching has always been associated with significant workloads. This is not new. Planning and assessment responsibilities have always been a critical aspect of a teacher's role, although requirements to report on students' progress and attainment were formalised following the 1988 Education Reform Act. Teachers generally enter teaching accepting that many of the planning, assessment and reporting responsibilities which they are required to undertake will need to be completed in their own time. Most teachers are aware that they will need to work during the evenings, weekends and school holidays. Most teachers are not afraid of hard work and they enjoy what they do. However, teaching is one of the few professions in which new teachers are required to demonstrate the same level of skill and undertake the same workload as more experienced colleagues (Tait, 2008).

Teacher workload becomes a problem when you do not manage to achieve and sustain a work–life balance. This is essential for good mental health, and poor work–life balance can lead to lack of sleep, exhaustion, stress, anxiety, depression and burnout. Teachers start to resent significant workloads when they feel that the work has no significant impact on their teaching and students' progress or attainment. This usually occurs when they are asked to carry out tasks for line managers or leadership teams which serve an accountability purpose or tasks which are required for no other reason than they are part of the school policy.

As a teacher, you will be required to work within school policies. However, when you complete a lesson plan or write feedback on a piece of student's work you should ask yourself the following question: *will this help my students to make more progress?* If the answer to this question is 'no' then you should reflect on why you are completing the task. Spending unnecessary time on lesson plans, marking and feedback is not a good investment of your time if it has no impact on your students. While you will need to plan for and assess learning, writing lengthy plans and overly detailed feedback does not guarantee student progress, particularly if students do not read the feedback. Consider ways in which you can reduce the time that you spend planning lessons and develop more productive ways of providing your students with feedback.

CRITICAL QUESTIONS

+ Why do you think that reducing teacher workload has recently become a policy priority?

+ What factors can result in unnecessary workload for teachers?

+ Are you able to identify any unnecessary workload that you currently have? Could you resist some of this and how might you go about doing this?

🖤 59 per cent of senior leaders, 29 per cent of teachers and 32 per cent of all education professionals work more than 51 hours a week on average.

🖤 58 per cent of all education professionals work more than 41 hours a week.

(ESP, 2018)

CASE STUDY

Amira was a headteacher in a primary school. She was aware that her teachers were spending too much time planning lessons and marking students' work and she felt that this was having a detrimental impact on their well-being. Amira decided to review the planning policy. The planning template was modified to include only the essential elements that were necessary to secure learning, and the requirement to word process planning and to hand it in for scrutiny on a weekly basis was lifted. The new planning template was optional and Amira allowed staff to develop their own planning formats that suited them if they chose not to use the template. She permitted teachers to hand-write their planning. The requirement to mark every single piece of work was lifted and instead teachers focused on sampling students' work during lessons to identify misconceptions. The focus shifted from providing students with written feedback on their work to verbal feedback during lessons. Misconceptions were addressed immediately in the lesson and became a focus for the next lesson. Students' books were sampled quickly after lessons to identify misconceptions and strengths and students were provided with whole-class generic feedback in the next lesson. Amira asked staff to design an assessment task for both

English and mathematics once every half-term. This was marked fully and students were provided with detailed written and verbal feedback on their performance in this task.

STUDENT BEHAVIOUR

Challenging behaviour and low-level disruption from students can result in teachers developing mental ill-health (Kryiacou, 2001). You may start to anticipate negative student behaviour in lessons and this can lead to anxiety. It is important to remember not to take the behaviour personally. Rarely is it personal. Negative behaviour is usually an attempt to communicate an unmet need. Sometimes it is a reaction to you as a symbol of authority rather than a reaction to you personally. Establishing positive relationships with all students by demonstrating unconditional positive regard towards them is one of the most effective ways of addressing student behaviour. Treating students with kindness, even in the face of hostility, is one of the best ways of demonstrating to them that you care. You will need to follow the school behaviour policy in addressing all student behaviour.

False allegations of misconduct on your part by students can also be extremely stressful. In these circumstances, you may need support from colleagues in your school, and your teaching union will also be able to offer you advice. It is important to remain calm and rational in these circumstances; if you have not committed an offence against a student, then it will be difficult for the student to prove it. However, this does not underplay the serious detrimental impact that false allegations can have on your own mental health.

PARENTAL EXPECTATIONS

Negative feedback from parents can result in teachers developing poor mental health. While schools can refuse to allow parents who are aggressive from entering the school premises, it is more difficult to stop parents from posting negative messages about teachers on social media sites. Parents may also contact you via email to provide negative feedback. If you feel that you are being bullied or harassed by a parent then you should discuss this immediately with your line manager. Your employers have a duty of care to you, as an employee, to protect you from harm. You should expect their support.

If a parent is upset and demands a meeting with you, do not feel obliged to meet them immediately, especially if you have a teaching commitment. Provide them with a time and, if you are anxious about the meeting, ask for a colleague to attend the meeting with you. Sit down with the parent and ask them to explain their concerns. Try not to interrupt them, maintain eye contact, avoid being defensive and note down some of the key points that they have made. When they have finished speaking, respond calmly to the points they have made and state clearly the facts of the case. Together with the parent, agree on the solutions which will address the concerns they have raised and explain how the case will be followed through or monitored. End on a positive note by thanking the parent for coming in to speak to you. If you feel threatened or intimidated, then you have a right to terminate the meeting.

EXTERNAL FACTORS

Teaching is all-encompassing. You will become used to writing a to-do list and not completing all the tasks on it. This can be stressful because many teachers like to be organised and on top of their workload. Most teachers manage to cope with the demands of their role. However, external factors can affect a teacher's ability to keep abreast of their commitments. The combination of work and family commitments can result in stress for teachers (Beltman et al, 2011). Examples of external factors which can affect a teacher's ability to cope with the day-to-day demands of their job include:

+ the death or illness of a family member or friend;

+ relationship problems;

+ financial problems, including debt;

+ housing problems;

+ parental commitments.

If your personal commitments unexpectedly increase, this can place pressure on you as a teacher. These commitments may take up all of your time outside of school, yet you are still required to complete your workload tasks which are an essential part of your job as a teacher. You may need to leave school earlier to attend to your personal commitments. You may need some flexibility in relation to your hours of work for a short period of time. You may need some adjustments to your teaching and other commitments to enable you to manage. The earlier that you talk to someone in school, the more responsive your colleagues can be in offering you advice and support.

CASE STUDY

Oliver was a mathematics teacher in a large secondary school. He was 27 and in a same-sex relationship. He was very committed and extremely hard-working but he hid something from his colleagues. His partner, Ian, was subjecting him to domestic abuse. Most of the abuse was emotional abuse but Ian had recently started to inflict physical and financial abuse on Oliver. Ian controlled every aspect of Oliver's life. He checked the messages on his phone, he told him what clothes he could wear and what he was allowed to eat, and he isolated him from his friends. Ian demanded that Oliver arrive home from school by 4.30pm each evening, thus placing Oliver under significant stress, especially if there were meetings after school.

Oliver did not want anyone to know about his situation at home. He felt ashamed of his situation and his confidence and self-worth had been eroded. He started to stay in school later into the evening so that he could avoid the situation at home. However, when Oliver did this, Ian subjected him to physical and verbal abuse.

One evening, after an argument, Ian refused to let Oliver go to sleep. He turned the music up to full volume so that Oliver could not go to sleep. When Oliver went to school the next morning he was exhausted. Over a period of time, the quality of Oliver's teaching had started to deteriorate. He could not concentrate on his school work and Ian refused to allow him to work at home. This was devastating to Oliver because he was a dedicated teacher; he loved working with his students but he did not know how to get help.

One day, Oliver arrived at school and broke down in front of his line manager. He could not cope any more. He was not able to concentrate, he had no confidence and he had started to become anxious in school. Oliver's line manager was supportive and was able to develop a plan to help Oliver.

CRITICAL QUESTIONS

+ In your opinion, was Oliver's decision to keep quiet about his personal circumstances the best decision?

+ If you had been Oliver's colleague, what would you have done to support him?

+ How effective was the school in supporting Oliver? What more could have been done to support him?

INTERNAL FACTORS

Personal factors can influence teacher well-being. Factors may include teachers' own health, confidence, self-worth, motivation, financial status and personal beliefs about their own competence.

Many factors contribute to teacher stress. Research demonstrates that negative student behaviour is associated with teacher burnout across all phases of education (Beltman et al, 2011). High workloads also increase teacher stress (Schonfeld, 2001). Paradoxically, although school climate impacts detrimentally on teacher stress, research has found that increased teacher stress may also negatively influence the school climate due to staff absenteeism and high rates of staff turnover (Grayson and Alvarez, 2008).

Of education professionals in 2017–18:

- 31 per cent experienced a mental health issue;

- 67 per cent described themselves as stressed;

- 80 per cent of senior leaders described themselves as stressed;

- 74 per cent were unable to switch off from work and relax;

- 76 per cent experienced behavioural, psychological or physical symptoms of mental ill-health;

- 57 per cent had considered leaving the sector over the previous two years;

- 72 per cent cited workload as the main reason for considering leaving their jobs;

- 65 per cent were not confident in disclosing mental ill-health to their employer;

- 35 per cent of senior leaders and 30 per cent of teachers believed that taking time off work due to mental ill-health would have a negative effect on working relationships with their colleagues.

(ESP, 2018)

Research demonstrates that the aspects of a positive school climate include an emphasis on academic achievement, positive relationships among students, teachers and between students and teachers, respect for all members of the school community, fair and consistent discipline policies, attention to safety issues, and family and community involvement (Wilson, 2004). Research has found that teachers are more productive, motivated and less stressed when leadership teams are supportive (Day, 2008).

SUMMARY

This chapter has explored some of the factors which contribute to teachers' mental ill-health. It has identified the actions which can be taken to reduce the risks of developing mental ill-health while acknowledging that some stress is inevitable, and that stress may not always be bad for you. This chapter has explained the importance of identifying when stress may be appropriate and when it is likely to become overwhelming. The importance of considering teacher workload has also been emphasised and strategies to reduce workload have been discussed.

CHECKLIST

This chapter has addressed:

✓ the extent of teacher mental ill-health;

✓ the factors which contribute to teachers' mental ill-health.

FURTHER READING

Cowley, A (2019) *The Wellbeing Toolkit: Sustaining, Supporting and Enabling School Staff*. London: Bloomsbury Education.

Morrison McGill, R (2016) *Mark. Plan. Teach: Save Time. Reduce Workload. Impact Learning*. London: Bloomsbury.

✚ CHAPTER 2

MANAGING YOUR CAREER JOURNEY

PROFESSIONAL LINKS

This chapter addresses the following:

🔗 Department for Education (DfE) (2018) *Addressing Teacher Workload in Initial Teacher Education (ITE): Advice for ITE Providers*. London: DfE.

🔗 Department for Education (DfE) (2019) *Early Career Framework*. London: DfE.

CHAPTER OBJECTIVES

By the end of this chapter you will understand:

+ some of the challenges that you might encounter during your Initial Teacher Training programme, your Newly Qualified Teacher (NQT) year and beyond;

+ ways of addressing these challenges so that you stay mentally healthy.

INTRODUCTION

This chapter outlines some of the feelings and emotions that you may experience while studying on a teacher training course, during your NQT year and beyond. It explains that you may feel overwhelmed at the beginning of your training programme but that it is important to acknowledge that there will be others who share these feelings. It also explains that you are also likely to experience challenges throughout your career, for example, as assessments and observations take place.

The chapter also introduces research from the Teacher Wellbeing Index (ESP, 2018) which highlights the key challenges associated with teaching. Additionally, the concept of imposter syndrome is described to illustrate how self-doubt can impede confidence. In this chapter, we argue that imposter syndrome is common in those beginning new jobs and careers and that it is important to recognise that you are not alone in experiencing these feelings. Practical ways of addressing and overcoming the challenges you may face are provided so that you can stay mentally healthy throughout your training and beyond.

THE INITIAL TEACHER TRAINING PHASE

This section considers specifically the challenges that you might experience during your Initial Teacher Training (ITT) phase and offers practical solutions for addressing these.

You might feel overwhelmed at the start of your teacher training programme and you will find that there are others who also feel exactly the same. If you are following a one-year programme of postgraduate training, you might quickly be introduced to lots of new content in the first few weeks of term. It might feel like you are literally being bombarded with content on a range of topics including, but not limited to, the curriculum, assessment, safeguarding, subject knowledge, behaviour management strategies, special educational needs and lesson planning. Don't be surprised if you initially start to feel slightly overwhelmed. You cannot learn everything there is to know about teaching in this way and not all of the information will be relevant to you at that specific time. Don't be afraid to 'park' some information in your long-term memory if you do not need it immediately. Focus on retaining what is needed to help you accomplish imminent challenges and be prepared to revisit content later on during your training.

With the best of intentions, teacher training providers ritually warn trainee teachers about how demanding the programme is going to be. This is often the first thing that trainees hear on day 1. Trainees are often informed about the demanding workload and they are warned that their social life will seriously suffer during the process of learning to be a teacher. It is not unusual for trainees to be told to expect that they will be working well into the night followed by very early starts the following morning. Although some of these warnings are usually well-intentioned, they can cause some trainees to feel stressed and anxious even before they have set foot inside a classroom. These messages can also be misleading because they can lead to trainees thinking that they should close down their social life and support networks for the duration of their training. In addition, they can result in trainees feeling guilty for taking time out.

It is important to remember that it is essential that you take some 'you' time during your training. It is crucial to make time for family and friends and it is essential to maintain a work–life balance. Having a social life is important for your well-being. Developing and sustaining social connections supports you to stay mentally healthy and finding time for physical activity improves your mental health. You should never feel guilty for taking time out and you should view this as a necessity rather than something to feel guilty about.

When you continually listen to people talking about the challenges associated with teaching, it is important to consider why teaching is a fantastic career choice. It provides you with an opportunity to make a positive difference to the lives of students. It is a richly rewarding career, especially when you see young people succeeding, gaining confidence and developing a positive sense of self. It provides you with intellectual stimulation and challenge and opportunities to be creative, both in your lesson delivery and in the way you solve problems. You will get to work with like-minded people as well as people who you find deeply frustrating and annoying. No two days are the same but you can go home every day knowing that you have made a difference, even if that difference is not visible to you at the time. Young people do not always value what you do for them at the time and even if they do, they do not always tell you that they value you. It is true, as a teacher, you change lives. There are not many careers that give you that same opportunity.

When you experience the challenges of teaching, you should remember all of these positives. As you start your training programme, it is a good idea to schedule all deadlines for tasks that you are required to complete and allocate time for completing these. Keeping an up-to-date well-organised diary will help to clear your mind because if you have written it down, then you will not forget to do it. It may be the first time that you have ever needed to keep a diary. Organising and managing your workload is a professional responsibility which you will need to master.

SELF-DOUBT

You may question your ability at any point during your training programme – *Can I do this? Will the students listen to me? Will they behave for me? What if I cannot answer their questions? Am I good enough? What if I fail?* Initially you might experience imposter syndrome, particularly when you stand in front of a class for the first time. The good news is that most people experience these types of feelings, particularly when they start a new job. It is not unusual to feel like this. The important thing to remember is that you are good enough because you have passed a rigorous selection process. You have also studied hard to gain the necessary academic qualifications to allow you to gain entry onto the programme. Many of your anxieties will be alleviated through thorough lesson preparation. As a trainee teacher, no-one should expect you to know everything. If you are unclear about something, you should ask for help and not see this as a failure on your part. If a student asks you a question that you cannot answer, praise them for asking a brilliant question and research the answer together with the class. They will respect you more for telling the truth. The difference between teaching and medicine is that students will not die if you do not know something, teach something incorrectly or if you have a bad lesson. Use these opportunities to reflect on your own development as a teacher and to help you grow further. In medicine, following an incorrect procedure can result in instant death so the consequences are far more serious. You have an opportunity in teaching to rectify your mistakes.

FITTING INTO SCHOOLS

You will naturally be excited to go into school to complete your periods of assessed teaching. However, it is useful to experience anxiety in new situations. You may be worried about whether you will 'fit in' to the overall school culture, whether you will experience a sense of belonging through being welcomed in and whether you will get on with your mentor and students. These concerns are all normal and after a few days in school you are likely to feel that you are just part of the furniture. If you have any concerns about your sense of belonging in a school, you should raise these with your programme tutor or school-based mentor earlier rather than later.

Most programmes provide opportunities for trainees to work in at least two schools. Moving schools can also trigger stress and anxiety. One way of addressing this is to visit the school prior to undertaking your block of assessed teaching so that you are familiar with the staff, policies and routines before you start.

It is important to invest time in establishing a positive relationship with your school-mentor. Mentors are often busy professionals who are responsible for balancing many other work-related commitments. Value their time but try not to over-depend on them. Although you may need greater support at the start of the programme, you should aim to develop your independence as you progress through it. Value their professional opinion and demonstrate to them that you are acting on their advice. Offer to support colleagues in school as well as being a recipient of support. Try to fit into the professional team that you are required to work with and radiate energy, enthusiasm and passion even when you are tired. Everyone is tired and it is worth remembering this. Value the time that people invest in you.

ASSIGNMENTS

If you are following an undergraduate or postgraduate programme of teacher training, you will almost certainly be required to complete academic assignments in addition to your school placements. You will be supported by your academic tutors who will help you to understand the assignment tasks and the required standards that you need to demonstrate. The obvious point to stress is to not leave everything until the last minute: this will create stress and anxiety. Start working on your assignment straightaway. Work on it little and often and you will be surprised at how quickly you can get it finished. The aim of producing a first draft is to get the assignment written, not to produce something that is perfect. Write it first and polish it up later. No author, however brilliant, can produce a perfect initial draft.

If you are new to academic writing in the social sciences, you will need to master specific skills including developing an argument, synthesising literature and critically analysing theory and research. You will also need to learn about academic referencing. If you are unsure, seek help. Many providers of teacher training offer academic skills support to help you reach the required standard. The more you write, the more you will improve.

Mark all of your deadlines on your calendar at the start of the academic year and allocate specific chunks of time to specific assignments. Working within small 'windows of time' can be more productive because it focuses your mind. If you know that you have three days to complete a task then it limits you to working within that time frame.

CRITICAL QUESTIONS

+ When might the 'pinch points' be during your ITT when you might experience greater stress and anxiety?
+ What other challenges might you experience during your ITT?

RESOURCES

Although you are likely to experience a range of challenges during your ITT, these can be offset through accessing resources which will support you in addressing the challenges. Your biggest and most important resource is the people around you. These include members of your family and friends. When you are experiencing stress or anxiety or doubting yourself, talking to others who you trust can really help. People who are close to you can provide you with practical advice, including coping strategies. They can also provide you with bucketloads of reassurance and emotional support. Learning to be a teacher is not just an intellectual process; it is an emotional roller-coaster of a journey in which you will experience highs as well as lows. You will have good days and bad days. Reaching out to others when you need support is not a sign of weakness. It is a sign of strength and it will help you to stay resilient.

There are others who can also offer you emotional support and practical advice. You have access to your programme tutors and leaders, school-based mentors and your peers who are training alongside you. You also have access to an online community of educators through social media. All of these people and networks can provide you with varied forms of support. It is important that you ask for support if you recognise that you need it.

It is not necessary for you to reinvent the wheel. Colleagues may have schemes of work, lesson plans and teaching resources that they are happy to share with you. This can help to reduce workload. Many teachers create and share resources via social networking platforms (for example, Twitter) and professional learning communities (for example, the *TES*).

When you experience challenges, it is useful to consider which resources you will draw upon to support you through these. The important thing to remember is that you do not need to solve all the problems alone. If you feel that you need help, ask for it and never view this as a sign of weakness. It is a sign of strength.

CASE STUDY

A trainee called Kieran was several weeks into his teacher training placement and was experiencing significant levels of anxiety. This anxiety was impacting on his emotional well-being. He had decided not to discuss this with his mentor as he felt he would be judged and seen as inexperienced and incompetent.

After two more weeks, Kieran became too anxious to attend his placement and was invited to meet with his mentor to discuss these feelings. In this meeting, Kieran explained that the source of his anxiety was the expectation that he be able to stand in front of a group of students despite being only five years older. The mentor explained that these feelings were common among some trainees. The mentor reassured Kieran that he was competent and able and had already passed a rigorous selection process to begin the programme. The mentor also buddied Kieran up with another trainee who had experienced similar feelings in recent weeks. This support enabled Kieran to resume some of his teaching commitments and gradually increase his classroom presence.

In a review meeting several weeks later, Kieran explained that he had associated his anxiety with incompetence and failure. He had not realised that other trainees had experienced similar emotions, feelings and challenges. He felt a sense of shame and isolation and this was only overcome through dialogue and support and through realising that his feelings were not personal and isolated. Kieran successfully completed his placement and now teaches on an ITT programme where he supports trainees by sharing his stories and experiences of his own training.

MANAGING THE ITT WORKLOAD

The Department for Education has produced guidance for schools and teacher training providers on reducing workload (DfE, 2018b). Providers of teacher training are advised through this guidance to reduce unnecessary workload for trainee teachers, particularly in relation to lesson planning, assessment and data management. School leaders should also be taking steps to reduce unnecessary workload for teachers.

Regardless of policy directives, you will be required, as a trainee, to adhere to the policies of your provider and the schools in which you are placed. Schools have vastly different policies on planning, assessment and teachers' use of time but there are steps that you can take to manage your own workload. These are outlined below.

+ Produce a daily 'to-do' list for the week.

+ Allocate specific 'windows of time' for specific tasks, including lesson planning and marking.

+ Prioritise tasks by completing the urgent tasks first.

+ Accept that you will never reach the end of your to-do list because unforeseen tasks will have to be completed.

+ Roll uncompleted tasks on to the next day or week.

+ Keep on top of your daily lessons preparation by organising resources for the next day's lessons into trays, box files, drawers or a different filing system so that the next day is prepared before you leave school.

+ Utilise school reprographic services for copying resources and send work to the service well in advance.

+ Utilise non-teaching time in school for planning and marking.

+ Plan lessons so that some lessons do not generate marking.

+ Make greater use of verbal and peer feedback in lessons, if appropriate and meaningful.

+ Sample students' books and identify generic feedback points. Start the next lesson by sharing your feedback with the class and use this as an opportunity to address misconceptions.

+ Reduce the quantity of written feedback on students' work.

+ Develop an assessment/recording system that enables you to address students' misconceptions and advance progress.

+ Keep recording systems simple, easy to complete and efficient to use.

+ Avoid spending time developing lesson resources that you will only use once.

+ Avoid planning lessons which require you to use too many resources which you will need to create.

+ Make use of departmental resources to support your planning.

CRITICAL QUESTIONS

+ How is your teacher training provider actively taking steps to reduce trainee workload?

+ How are your school leaders actively taking steps to reduce unnecessary workload for staff?

MANAGING STUDENT BEHAVIOUR

Student behaviour is one of the things that keeps trainee teachers (and qualified teachers) awake at night. You might worry about losing control of a class or how you will manage low-level disruption and more challenging behaviour. Student behaviour can disrupt teaching and impact negatively on learning. It is one of the factors that results in teachers leaving the profession.

Firstly, it is important to recognise that students 'test out' all new teachers to see how far they can 'push them'. Rarely is poor behaviour personal and it is likely that most disruption will be low level. Set out your expectations clearly with a new class. Do not be afraid to issue rewards and sanctions in line with school policy and never ignore poor behaviour. Read the school's behaviour policy and adhere to it. Use verbal and non-verbal cues including facial expressions, body posture and eye contact with students who are demonstrating inappropriate behaviour. Consistently apply sanctions in line with school policy and praise good behaviour. Be consistent and insistent. Once you have communicated clear expectations, you will soon be able to relax with your students.

Secondly, ask for help if you are struggling. Again, this is not a sign of weakness. Talk to your school-based mentors, provider tutors and other colleagues in school. You should also consider asking colleagues to share behaviour strategies with you on professional online networks.

Thirdly, remember that the issues are not unique to you. Most teachers experience these problems on a daily basis. Reflect on your practice regularly, develop new strategies and evaluate their effectiveness.

Finally, use your professional development time to observe more experienced teachers managing behaviour. Notice how they reward good behaviour, sanction poor behaviour and apply techniques to de-escalate problems. Try to stay calm, even in challenging situations, and remember that you are the adult. There are multiple complex reasons for poor behaviour and establishing positive relationships with students will prevent much poor behaviour from occurring in the first place. Start each new lesson afresh and always believe that students can improve their behaviour.

CRITICAL QUESTIONS

+ What strategies are outlined in your school behaviour policy?
+ What are the advantages and disadvantages of the use of rewards and sanctions for managing student behaviour?

MANAGING RELATIONSHIPS

Developing relationships with your ITT mentor is essential, not only for your sanity, but because they are responsible for assessing you. Managing relationships is important in teaching because it is a job that involves working with people, and people can be unpredictable. It is fantastic when you hit it off with your mentor straightaway. However, with some mentors you may have to tread carefully and it may be more difficult to establish a relationship with them.

WHAT IF THINGS GO WRONG?

If things go wrong for you, it is upsetting but it is not the end of the world. If you do not pass a placement or an assignment there will usually be a resit opportunity. The key thing is to determine what went wrong so that you can ensure that this is not repeated on the second attempt. Ask for help from your networks and talk to people who are close to you about how you feel. Your school-based mentor or provider tutor is also likely to be able to offer you feedback and guidance. You should accept any opportunities to meet with these staff and you should consider and address their advice moving forward. It is important to remember that these staff are usually experienced and knowledgeable and that any guidance they offer can be invaluable even though it can sometimes be difficult to discuss your areas for development. To support your confidence, it can be helpful to reflect on the successes and strengths of your placement so far. The worst thing you can do in these situations is to cut yourself off from people. It is worth remembering that you will not be the first person this has happened to and you will certainly not be the last.

THE NQT PHASE

This section considers specifically the challenges that you might experience during your NQT year and offers practical solutions for addressing these.

There is limited research into the early professional development of new teachers (Totterdell et al, 2004, 2005). Existing literature demonstrates that the induction process for NQTs has been a cause for concern for several years (Haggarty and Postlethwaite, 2012). One suggested reason for this is the apparent discontinuity of experiences in the transition from ITT to the induction year (Hobson et al, 2007). It has been argued that there is little evidence of a staged, progressive induction process through which knowledge and skills are developed over time (Harrison, 2001). Additionally, models of support tend to adopt a deficit approach by targeting support on addressing weaknesses in teacher performance (Harrison, 2001; Haggarty and Postlethwaite, 2012) rather than developing teachers' skills further to support them in becoming more effective.

The Early Career Framework (DfE, 2019) for NQTs is operational from September 2020. It provides a staged process of professional development for all new teachers over a two-year period and provides a guarantee of additional non-class contact time for professional development (5 per cent) and mentor support in the second year of teaching.

FINDING A SCHOOL

In the rush to find employment, it is easy to apply for jobs in all schools within a specific region that have advertised posts. However, accepting a job for the sake of securing employment may not be in your best interests in the long run and you might end up working in a school and being deeply unhappy.

It is important to remember that applying for a job is an opportunity for you to select the right school for you as well as an opportunity for the school to select the right candidate. Try to visit the school during the working day to get a 'feel' for it. Often, it is possible to sense the culture within a school within the first few minutes. Do as much research as you can to find out about the school. Look at the school website, read the latest Ofsted report and during an initial visit ask the senior staff what the best thing is about working there and what support will be provided for NQTs. Ask yourself:

+ Is this a happy place to work?

+ Will I enjoy working here?

+ Is the culture positive?

+ Are the students happy?

It is important that you select a school which will support you to thrive during your NQT year. This is a critical stage in your development as a teacher and you will need support, guidance and encouragement to fulfil your potential. Ideally, you want to be employed in a school in which it is acceptable to ask for help if you encounter personal or professional challenges.

BUILDING RELATIONSHIPS WITH YOUR CLASSES

As an NQT you will be keen to establish positive relationships with your students. Students are more likely to thrive when they have a teacher who is motivated, enthusiastic, approachable and cares about them. However, you initially need to establish clear expectations for behaviour so that boundaries are established from the outset. Students generally respond well to rules and expectations, and the school behaviour policy will guide you. It is reasonable to expect students to 'test' you at first, but they generally adapt their behaviour when they realise that you will not tolerate inappropriate behaviour. Try to keep your cool, stay calm but be consistent and insistent. Once your expectations are established, you will be able to relax with your students but if you start off without clear expectations, it is more difficult to impose them subsequently.

It is important to learn students' names as quickly as possible. This can be more difficult in secondary schools if you are teaching hundreds of students each week. A seating plan will help.

BUILDING A RELATIONSHIP WITH YOUR NQT MENTOR

Your mentor plays a critical role in your development as a teacher during your first year of teaching. Effective mentors provide NQTs with constructive feedback on their teaching and offer practical guidance. They also provide opportunities to support the professional development of NQTs. In addition, high-quality mentors pay close attention to the pastoral care needs of NQTs, particularly in cases where new teachers may also be experiencing personal difficulties. Good mentors provide NQTs with an appropriate level of challenge and offer them support to help them to achieve their targets.

Establishing an effective relationship with your mentor should be your priority. When relationships break down this can result in NQTs experiencing stress, anxiety and depression. These factors can impact detrimentally on the quality of their teaching. Value the experience of your mentor, thank them for their feedback and demonstrate to them that you have acted on their advice. Try not to be too demanding of their time by respecting the fact that they may have other responsibilities on top of mentoring. Aim to work autonomously and ask for advice when you feel that you need it.

One strategy for developing effective relationships with your mentor is to fully immerse yourself in the life of the school. By offering to participate in extra-curricular activities and volunteering to take on responsibilities, you are demonstrating your commitment to the school. It is important to show that you are prepared to give something back to the school as a way of demonstrating your appreciation for the support you are being given.

Mentors will be impressed by you if you show commitment, enthusiasm and hard work. You will also create a good impression if you demonstrate that you are organised and efficient at undertaking your responsibilities. Take control of your own professional learning by demonstrating that you are able to identify development needs and able to suggest ways in which you might address these. During your first year of teaching, good mentors will not expect perfection but they will be looking for dedication, drive and determination to succeed. Good mentors will nurture you, but they cannot do the work for you. Ultimately, you have to be willing to put in the effort so that you can be the best you can be.

Research has demonstrated the following:

The role of the mentor as pivotal during the NQT year was emphasised by the participants in this study. They [NQTs] emphasised the importance of having access to both formal and informal support from their mentor and the necessity for constructive feedback and target setting.

(Glazzard and Coverdale, 2018, p 96)

However, it is also important to recognise that other members of staff in the school can provide you with valuable networks of support (Glazzard and Coverdale, 2018). Good mentors will encourage you to gain support from members of the wider school community. A mentor cannot be an expert in all aspects of pedagogy but they can signpost you to colleagues who have relevant expertise. You should make the most of the opportunity to learn from others and this will take some pressure off the mentor.

BEING ACCOUNTABLE DURING YOUR NQT YEAR

Being accountable for students' progress and attainment is probably the greatest source of anxiety for many NQTs. During your ITT you were never truly accountable for students' progress, even though this is stated in the Teachers' Standards (DfE, 2011). The qualified teacher whose class(es) you are covering is responsible ultimately for students' learning. As an NQT, the accountability rests with you.

Knowing that you are accountable for students' learning can result in stress and anxiety, particularly if your students make less than expected progress during the year. Monitoring the progress of your students regularly throughout the year through using reliable assessment tools (eg tests or quizzes) is a good way of identifying quickly which students need additional intervention to make greater progress. It is important to assess students not only at the end of units of work, but also at the start of units of work and throughout them to identify gaps in know-ledge, skills and misconceptions. These formative assessments can then be used to modify your subsequent teaching and to help you iden-tify those students who need specific interventions. It is also important to assess students not only immediately after a unit of work but also several weeks or months after a unit has been completed to help you identify if subject content has been retained and understood.

Try not to be too anxious if your students make less than expected pro-gress. There will usually be good explanations for under-achievement and some of the factors may be outside of your control. You will need to be able to explain a student's under-achievement but an effective lead-ership team should also acknowledge the influence of external factors that result in this.

Sfard and Prusak (2005) identified two types of identity: actual identity, which refers to a personal identity, and desired (or assigned) identity, which refers to an identity which is imposed on the individual by others. Learning to be a teacher involves a considerable degree of identity work. New teachers may hold personal values and beliefs about the kind of teacher they want to be, but these may conflict with the identity which is assigned to them. The assigned identity indicates the type of teacher that they must be in order to survive. Typically, this is a teacher who can raise academic attainment. While this aim is laudable, it is problematic because it can result in other values being compromised.

MANAGING NEW PROFESSIONAL EXPERIENCES DURING YOUR NQT YEAR

During your first year of teaching you will have to do certain tasks for the first time. This can be frightening and lead to stress, anxiety and panic! Examples include:

+ leading an assembly;

+ organising an educational visit;

+ running a parents' evening;

+ preparing your class for sports day;

+ inputting assessment data into data monitoring systems.

One way to manage these stressful situations is to ask for help or to observe other colleagues who are also engaged in these activities. Don't be afraid to ask for advice, especially if you are doing something for the first time, and don't try to make it perfect. The more you do something, the better you will be at doing it.

MANAGING RELATIONSHIPS WITH PARENTS

Secondary school teachers have limited contact with parents but primary teachers usually have to meet and greet parents each day. Parents are also usually more involved in their child's primary education than their secondary education.

It can be daunting as an NQT opening the classroom door to greet parents. Most parents will trust you to do your job but others will be more demanding. Some parents may constantly complain about you and this can undermine your confidence and lead to stress and anxiety. The following points might be useful in establishing boundaries and effective relationships with parents.

+ Always insist that they make an appointment to see you after school rather than trying to talk to you first thing in the morning, particularly if they wish to make a complaint or are unhappy about something. This will provide you with valuable thinking time.

+ If you feel intimidated by a parent and they wish to meet you, reserve the right to meet them with a more experienced member of staff.

+ Do not reply to parent emails late at night. Manage their expectations by answering emails during the working day.

+ Communicate with them regularly via newsletters so they are aware of the latest initiatives and events.

+ Communicate successes with them regularly, for example when a student has impressed you or made you proud.

+ Listen to their concerns, acknowledge their feelings, try not to be defensive and agree a way forward.

PROGRESSING THROUGH YOUR CAREER

This section considers specifically the challenges that you might experience beyond your NQT year and offers practical solutions for addressing these.

In June 2018, the Department for Education published its School Workforce in England analysis. Its headline figures provide a useful summary of teacher recruitment and retention in England between 2016 and 2017, showing that:

- the number of FTE (full-time equivalent) teachers in all schools fell by 1.2 per cent (from 457,200 to 451,900);

- the number of FTE nursery and primary teachers fell by 0.6 per cent (from 222,400 to 221,200);

- the number of FTE secondary teachers fell by 1.9 per cent (from 208,200 to 204,200).

    At the same time, the analysis summarised the rate of change in student numbers. This included:

- the rate of increase in nursery and primary student numbers slowing, with the figure stabilising in 2019;

- the rate of increase in secondary student numbers rising, with this projection expected until 2025.

(DfE, 2018a)

DOING YOUR BEST

Bethune (2018) argues the case for the 'good-enough teacher'. These are teachers who do their best to care for their students and do all they can to provide them with a good education. They try to make their lessons interesting and develop within their students a love of learning (Bethune, 2018). They focus on meeting students' physical, emotional and spiritual needs and on their happiness but sometimes they get it wrong and their lessons may be uninspiring.

Bethune makes an important point. It is fine to be 'good enough'. You cannot be outstanding all the time. No teacher will have the time or energy to deliver consistently inspiring lessons. It is acceptable to teach lessons that are consistently good. Take the pressure off yourself. No-one should expect you to be consistently outstanding and when you are tired, your performance will naturally dip.

Try not to see mistakes as failures. All teachers make mistakes and some mistakes are pretty big! Use mistakes as learning opportunities and do not beat yourself up about them. Accept that you will make mistakes within your teaching and wider professional practice and accept that you cannot be outstanding all the time. Doing your best is all anyone can ask for. If you have good relationships with your colleagues, they will forgive you for your mistakes and good colleagues will not hold these against you.

PERFECTIONISM

Teachers who are perfectionists demonstrate the following traits.

+ They aim to be graded consistently outstanding.

+ They spend a disproportionate amount of time planning lessons.

+ They work very long hours.

+ They aim to complete all of their jobs on their 'to-do' list.

+ They view their mistakes as failures, resulting in disappointment.

+ They compare their lessons to others.

(Bethune, 2018)

Many teachers are naturally perfectionists. They may have consistently experienced academic success throughout their lives and may strive for this in their own teaching. The problem here is that academic success does not guarantee that someone will be an excellent teacher. Nevertheless, perfectionists will strive for excellence in everything they do.

Although perfectionism can be admirable, it can also result in burnout and attrition from the profession. This is because perfectionism cannot be sustained over a long period of time. There will be times during the year when you will have to cut corners in order to survive. At certain points in the year, you will be swamped with multiple jobs which all need to be completed and to achieve this you will need to allocate less time to them than you would normally devote to them. You may need to cut down on your planning and marking, and usually this will not have any negative impact on your students. Perfectionist teachers may spend time on tasks which do not make any difference to students' outcomes. It is necessary to cut corners sometimes in order to survive and you must never feel guilty about this. The reality is that at times it is impossible to do the job without cutting corners.

You complete your planning so that you know what you are teaching. There is no need to write out a full script in preparation for a lesson if two or three bullet points will enable you to teach the lesson successfully. Although word-processed planning may look neat and tidy, a few handwritten scribbly notes can be just as effective. Stop wasting time on things that do not make a difference to students' learning. Before you write something down or fill in some paperwork, consider whether it is absolutely essential for your students or whether it is a task just for the sake of doing a task. If the latter applies, don't waste time on it. View your mistakes as a normal part of learning to be a teacher rather than as failures. Strip away unnecessary stresses (Bethune, 2018) and focus on doing only what is necessary to secure the best outcomes for your students. The pursuit of perfectionism will only make you exhausted. Be 'good enough' (Bethune, 2018) rather than being a perfectionist.

CHALLENGES IN YOUR TEACHING CAREER

The Teacher Wellbeing Index (ESP, 2018) identified the key challenges associated with teaching. These included:

+ high workloads;

+ unnecessary paperwork;

+ poor student behaviour;

+ long hours;

+ pressure.

Although it is likely that you will experience all of these challenges, there may be other challenges that are associated with training to be a teacher. These are outlined below.

The well-being see-saw (Dodge et al, 2012) demonstrates how optimum well-being is achieved when challenges are balanced with resources. The model is shown in Figure 2.1.

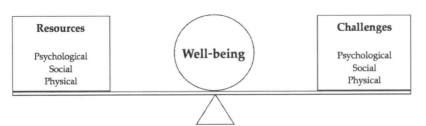

Figure 2.1 The well-being see-saw.

(Dodge et al, 2012)

The model positions well-being as being stable only if an individual has the psychological, social and physical resources that are needed in order to meet the individual's psychological, social and physical challenges (Dodge et al, 2012).

As a trainee, you will experience different challenges as you progress through the programme. Each time you meet one of these challenges, the well-being see-saw is drawn into a state of imbalance as you may not yet have mastered the resources that are required to over-come the challenges you will experience. When you experience new challenges and do not yet have the resources to draw from, the see-saw dips, along with your well-being (Dodge et al, 2012). The same is also true vice-versa.

As a trainee, it is important to acknowledge that your well-being is not static or stable. It is normal to experience different feelings and emotions and at times you will feel challenged. Thus, your well-being may tilt or shift depending on external factors and on your own experiences. In these times it is essential to identify the resources that you have available and to establish when it feels appropriate to ask for additional support or guidance.

MANAGING PERSONAL COMMITMENTS

Teaching is a demanding job that requires commitment, dedication and time. However, teaching is a career and should enhance your life rather than replace it. It is essential in teaching that you remain organised and up-to-date with your commitments and responsibilities; however, it is essential to plan and dedicate time to your personal commitments including your family, body and mind. Exercise and hobbies must not be lost or given up at the expense of your commitment to teaching. Many trainees and teachers also have caring commitments to children and family members. You must be able to accept that your to-do list will never be empty and that you will need to move tasks to future days and weeks in order to safeguard time for your personal commitments. This is essential in order for you to maintain a work–life balance and you should not feel guilty for managing your teaching commitments based on urgency and importance.

CASE STUDY

Lara, a teacher with caring responsibilities, had been finding it increasingly challenging to balance the demands of her personal and professional commitments. Lara was becoming increasingly anxious about these demands and decided to discuss them with the school leadership team. Lara contacted the Education Support Partnership, which is a charity dedicated to improving the health and well-being of school staff. The charity provided a trained counsellor who could discuss Lara's personal circumstances and offer tailored and confidential advice independently of the school.

The school discussed the situation with Lara. It was agreed that Lara's weekly teaching commitment would be reduced for a period of time. Through reducing the weekly teaching commitment, Lara had less planning and marking to complete and consequently there was a reduction in workload. This enabled Lara to balance her personal and professional commitments.

Glazzard and Rose (2019) found that teachers were just able to cope with their professional commitments. However, they experienced a tipping point when things went wrong in their personal lives. Examples include the death of a parent or child, family illness, divorce or separation. These external factors impacted on teachers' abilities to meet their professional commitments and resulted in them developing mental ill-health. They found that teacher 'presenteeism', where teachers continued to work but they were not focused on their jobs due to external factors, this led to a reduction in teaching quality and had a negative impact on students' learning.

The Teacher Voice Omnibus (2016), conducted by the National Foundation for Educational Research (NFER), surveyed over 1800 teachers from nearly 1600 schools in the maintained sector. The research demonstrates some interesting statistics in relation to teachers' perceptions of student behaviour.

- 75 per cent of respondents reported that behaviour in their school was good or very good.

- 17 per cent of respondents reported that behaviour in their school was acceptable.

- A greater percentage of respondents in primary schools (41 per cent) felt that behaviour in their school was very good compared to only 24 per cent of respondents from secondary schools.

- The percentage of senior leaders who felt behaviour in their school was very good was higher (48 per cent) than the percentage of classroom teachers who felt the same (21 per cent).

(NFER, 2016)

SUMMARY

This chapter has explored some of the feelings and emotions that you may experience at different stages of your teaching career. The chapter has also explained that although you may feel overwhelmed at specific points in your career, it is important to acknowledge that there will be others who share these feelings. Additionally, the chapter has introduced research from the Teacher Wellbeing Index (ESP, 2018) which highlighted the key challenges associated with teaching. The concept of imposter syndrome has been described to illustrate how self-doubt can impede confidence, and practical ways of addressing and overcoming the challenges you may face have been provided.

CHECKLIST

This chapter has addressed:

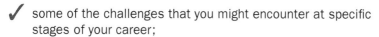 some of the challenges that you might encounter at specific stages of your career;

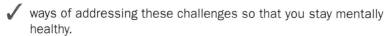 ways of addressing these challenges so that you stay mentally healthy.

FURTHER READING

Gumbrell, D (2019) *LIFT!: Going Up If Teaching Gets You Down* (Practical Teaching). St Albans: Critical Publishing.

Paramour, Z (2018) *How to Be an Outstanding Primary Middle Leader* (Outstanding Teaching). London: Bloomsbury Education.

✚ CHAPTER 3

MANAGING YOUR WORKLOAD

PROFESSIONAL LINKS

This chapter addresses the following:

Department for Education (DfE) (2018) *Addressing Teacher Workload in Initial Teacher Education (ITE): Advice for ITE Providers.* London: DfE.

Office for Standards in Education (Ofsted) (2019) *The Education Inspection Framework.* Manchester: Ofsted.

CHAPTER OBJECTIVES

By the end of this chapter you will understand:

+ some of the factors contributing to teachers disliking their jobs and to teachers' poor mental health;

+ a range of practical strategies that you can use to support your own workload in relation to planning, assessment and data management.

INTRODUCTION

This chapter outlines some of the challenges you may experience in relation to your own workload. It draws on recent research in order to support you in understanding how teacher workload can impact on positive mental health. The chapter also outlines and explains a range of additional factors known to impact on teacher well-being, satisfaction and mental health. As well as teacher workload, these factors include school climate, life satisfaction, responsibility, relationships, autonomy and opportunities for personal growth. Critical questions are asked to support your self-reflection and encourage you to think about these factors in relation to your own professional practice.

The chapter then offers a range of practical strategies to enable you to address and overcome some of the common challenges experienced by teachers. Specifically, the chapter draws on key elements of professional practice including planning, assessment and data management. For each of these, a range of common challenges are identified and discussed. In response to each of these, practical advice is offered to enable you to reduce your workload while maintaining your impact on students' progress. It is hoped that this will support you in staying mentally healthy both throughout your training and beyond.

WORKLOAD IS ONLY PART OF THE PROBLEM

Although many teachers object to bureaucracy and completing paperwork 'just for the sake of it', most are hard-working, highly committed and willing to complete the workload tasks associated with their roles, providing that they can see the purpose of the workload. Most teachers go into teaching with their eyes wide open. They anticipate a high workload and they know that this comes with the territory.

In 2018, the Teacher Wellbeing Index (ESP, 2018) demonstrated that workload and unnecessary paperwork were the biggest factors which contributed to teachers disliking their jobs. However, despite this national survey, a body of academic research in this area suggests that other factors also contribute to poor teacher mental health.

Research demonstrates that multiple factors impact on teacher well-being, including school climate (Gray et al, 2017). A negative school climate can lead to high rates of teacher absenteeism and staff turnover (Grayson and Alvarez, 2008). Conversely, a positive school climate results in better teacher engagement, higher levels of commitment and increased staff and student self-esteem and well-being (Gray et al, 2017). Teacher well-being is influenced by factors such as life satisfaction and personal happiness (hedonic perspective) and positive psychological functioning. Teachers are able to demonstrate positive psychological functioning when they are able to form good interpersonal relationships with others, have a sense of autonomy/agency and competence, and when they are provided with opportunities for personal growth (Harding et al, 2019).

CRITICAL QUESTIONS

+ How does school climate influence teacher workload?

+ What are the factors that might contribute to a positive school climate?

+ What are the factors that might contribute to a negative school climate?

+ Why might some school leaders restrict the autonomy/agency of teachers?

THE ISSUE OF WORKLOAD AND TEACHER MENTAL HEALTH

High workloads can result in exhaustion and burnout. However, research by Glazzard and Rose (2019) showed the following:

Whilst it is generally assumed that poor mental health – such as stress and anxiety – in teachers is caused largely by the pressure of work alone – particularly increasing workloads – this study found that this is not necessarily the case; it is only part of the story. It would appear [that] it is a combination of both personal life and professional pressures... Indeed, it would seem to be a finely balanced tightrope that teachers walk daily. When life and work are both running smoothly most teachers can and do cope. But when one or the other becomes more challenging than usual – for example, a breakdown in a personal relationship or sickness amongst the family or the pressure of SATs or assessment periods – that is when the difficulties arise. As one teacher observed: 'most people will be ok if everything else is ok in their life'.

(Glazzard and Rose, 2019, p 23)

The issue with workload is that most teachers are perfectionists. They generally want to complete every single workload-related task to the highest standard and many teachers feel guilty about cutting corners. You will quickly realise that it is not possible to achieve perfection in everything you do. You will have to prioritise and you will certainly have to take shortcuts in order to survive. There are simply too many jobs to do and not enough hours in the day to do them in to complete everything to a high standard. You must never feel guilty about this. It really is the only way to survive. You will have to accept that 'good enough' is 'good enough'. Focus your time and energy on workload-related tasks which will have the greatest impact on your students and complete all the other tasks as quickly as possible. Exhausted and burnt-out teachers are no good for students. Put your energies into tasks which matter and complete these to the best of your ability. Prioritise the tasks which you need to do and put the others further down the to-do list.

CONTROLLING WORKLOAD

Sometimes you will feel as if your workload is spiralling out of control. You will be faced with so many jobs to do and insufficient time to do them in. You will also hit 'hot spots' during the year when your workload is disproportionally high and there will be times when your workload is lighter. You are likely to find that workload is higher during assessment periods or when you are writing reports and preparing for parents' evenings.

Sometimes we experience greater stress when we think about all the work that we have to do. The to-do list keeps growing and our stress levels increase. The important thing to remember is that you cannot always complete every task on your list and you have to decide which tasks to prioritise. Even if you do manage to complete every task, you might not be able to complete them to the standard to which you aspire. The best way of tackling a to-do list is to make a start on the tasks rather than spending time thinking about how long the list is.

You will need to decide how much time you can allocate to each task. This is important because a single task could take you 30 minutes or two hours depending on what allocation of time you assign to it. Some teachers actually work with a timer at the side of them. They allocate a specific time to a task, start the timer and stop the task when the time is up. Sometimes it is more productive to work in shorter chunks of time. Spending too long on a task can be counter-productive and can lead to time being wasted. Working intensively on a task in a really focused way for a specific period of time can be really helpful. If you have 30 books to mark and only have an hour to mark them in, you know that you need to have marked 15 books after half an hour. Although this may seem like a military way of working, it can help you to be more efficient. Working within shorter 'windows of time' can really support you to get things done and it is also important to allocate time for relaxation.

Some teachers wait for a large block of time to tackle their to-do list. Then they experience frustration when this time never arrives. It is always more effective to work 'little and often'. If you have 20 minutes, make a start on a task, then stop and finish it at another time. You may be the sort of person who cannot work like this. You may need to start and finish one task before moving on to the next task rather than working on several tasks at the same time. We all work differently and we have to find a way of working that suits us.

If you have work-related tasks to do at weekends or during school holidays, decide what your optimum time is for working. Some teachers prefer to wake up early and work first thing in the morning. Others are more productive when they work in the afternoons, evenings or during the night. You will know your own body best and therefore you will be able to identify your optimum working time. Obviously during school time, you will have no choice about when you work!

Another way of controlling your workload is to refuse tasks. Obviously, some tasks are essential and you will not be able to refuse them. However, you will find that your workload spirals out of control if you simply say 'yes' to everything. Do not feel guilty about saying 'no' to people, especially if colleagues are trying to pass their workload on to you. This does happen. Although you may feel that it is rude to refuse a task, you should ask yourself this question:

When I say yes to someone, who am I saying no to?

This should put things into perspective for you. If you agree to do a job for someone, then you are ultimately agreeing to spending time on that task when you could be spending time on a different task. Also, it is important to remember who your line manager is and your objectives that were agreed during your last appraisal. Work strategically by only agreeing to tasks which will contribute to you achieving your annual objectives. Make sure that you are working on tasks that you have agreed with your line manager and try not to take on additional tasks which take you away from those that you have agreed.

Sometimes an appropriate response is to say this:

At the moment I do not have the time to do that task to the standard that I would want to do it.

Or you might say this:

I cannot do it right now but I can do it next week/month/term/year.

The problem is that most teachers want to please others. They spend all of their time saying 'yes' to other people and this results in them experiencing stress. It is acceptable to say 'no' to something, particularly if it is not part of your agreed objectives, not part of your role and not a priority for you. Try to get better at saying 'no' and try to find ways of expressing this without upsetting people. It is sometimes acceptable to refuse tasks from your line manager providing that you have solid justification for doing this.

CRITICAL QUESTIONS

+ How do you control your workload?
+ What factors result in workload spiralling out of control?

MANAGING YOUR PLANNING

Planning is crucial to effective teaching and learning and plays a critical role in supporting students' progress. However, too often, teachers feel obliged to 'reinvent the wheel' in order to ensure high expectations of lesson planning, resources and content. Often, high-quality resources are available from colleagues, and may include textbooks, and it is important that these are used to support teaching and reduce your workload.

It is important to acknowledge and recognise the difference between *a lesson plan* and *your lesson planning*. Too often, the term *planning* is used to refer to the production of lesson plans. These documents can evidence your thinking and may be requested by your school or training provider. However, this evidence functions only by proxy and a lesson plan on its own does not support student progress. While you will need to comply with school policy, it is worth considering the resources and time that you are committing to the production of the lesson plan and whether this commitment is reducing your capacity to focus on the crucial thinking that underpins your planning approaches and decisions. It is important to remember that your planning approaches are highly likely to impact students' progress whereas the production of the lesson plan itself is less likely to. The process of producing a lesson plan is significantly distinct from the decisions you have made in relation to planning, and it is critical to remember this distinction when allocating your time. It is therefore essential to ask for early clarification from your school in relation to their policy for evidencing your planning. Prior to this discussion, it is worth considering some key questions.

+ Can lesson plans be handwritten instead of needing to be produced digitally?

+ Can I change or amend a lesson plan by hand without needing to re-type or re-print it? Can I cross things out and re-write things?

+ Can I use a format I feel comfortable with? Can this be a blank piece of paper or some sticky notes?

+ Instead of needing to create a lesson plan, can I submit my annotated resources to support and evidence my thinking?

+ If I plan my lessons by making notes and annotating my PowerPoint, do I still need to type these thoughts up and create a lesson plan?

+ Can I use my own pro-forma? Can I amend the school pro-forma?

+ Do I need to produce lesson plans if they do not support my thinking or impact student progress?

Although internal policy may require the production of lesson plans, these questions may support you in ensuring that lesson plans are only being produced where there is a rationale and a clear link to student progress. Lesson plans and your lesson planning must both link directly to students' progress and not the satisfaction or appeasement of an observer or outside organisation.

As a teacher, it is important to structure and organise your resources so that these can be recalled easily in the future. It is also helpful to collaborate with colleagues both in the school and through online subject forums to build up or access established banks of readily available resources. These may be organised by subject, course or topic and it is important to consider the requirements of your own curriculum when deciding how to structure and store existing resources. You may also find it helpful to request that departmental or staff meeting time is used to support co-planning or collaboration. This allows staff to work together and support the introduction of, for example, a new topic, unit or module rather than one member of staff taking full responsibility for a new or reformed curriculum area.

CRITICAL QUESTIONS

+ What strategies have you found useful to help you manage your planning-related workload?

+ Where might you have committed time, unnecessarily, to the creation of resources or lesson material?

+ What does the latest Ofsted guidance say about planning?

MANAGING ASSESSMENT

Assessment is crucial to effective teaching and learning. Marking and feedback provides an opportunity for teachers and students to interact. It allows teachers to acknowledge and check students' work and make decisions about what needs to be done next in order to secure progress. However, in some cases, there is a belief that effective teachers must spend hours marking students' work. Writing pages of feedback does not make a teacher effective, nor does the quantity of marking given to students. The quantity of feedback must never be confused with the quality of feedback. Marking practices that do not impact on students' progress will simply waste teachers' and students' time and must therefore stop.

Your school is likely to have its own policy in relation to assessment and this may outline expectations in relation to the frequency, type and volume of marking and feedback. It is important that your marking and feedback is consistent with this policy. Your school policy may recognise and acknowledge subject- or age-specific requirements in relation to assessment in order to ensure that the policy is effective in promoting learning and catering to the needs of all students and all subjects.

In 2016, the government published the results of its independent report on eliminating unnecessary workload relating to marking. The principles of this report stated that all marking should be manageable, mean-ingful and motivating (DfE, 2016a). Manageable assessment policies should be clear that marking must be proportionate, and they should consider the frequency and complexity of written feedback as well as the effectiveness in terms of teachers' time in relation to workload. However, teachers may have little autonomy and flexibility in relation to how manageable their school's assessment policy is. Despite this, there are many different approaches a teacher can take to ensure that their marking is meaningful and motivating.

Oral feedback enables teachers to react quickly to students and their needs and can be given regularly and interactively throughout lessons. Oral feedback can be very effective as it can be given during or very quickly after an episode of learning. This increases opportunities for dialogue and communication, and it ensures that students understand the feedback they have been given. This enables them to respond to and action feedback instantly rather than wait between or across sequences of lessons. This type of feedback can be direct (targeted at individuals and groups) or indirect (where others may be listening and encourages reflection on the dialogue taking place). Oral feedback is effective when it provides meaningful guidance and advice that allows students to recognise their strengths and respond to their areas of development in a timely and specific manner. Using oral feedback to support students' progress can significantly reduce the time spent giving written feedback, which can reduce workload or free up time for teachers to focus on other tasks.

Live marking can also be used to reduce teachers' marking workload outside of lessons while still ensuring that students have access to regular and meaningful feedback. Live marking can involve a teacher marking with an individual student during lessons or it can involve marking work in front of a group of students using a visualiser. During live marking, teachers should consider highlighting students' work to indicate areas of improvement though corrections should not be made by the teacher as this ensures that the onus remains with the student and does not become the teacher's responsibility. Furthermore, live marking enables teachers to identify common areas of improvement among students and enables instant feedback to be given to individual students or groups of students.

Book sampling can be used by teachers to identify common strengths and areas of development. Prior to sampling students' work, teachers should establish how they will record strengths and areas of development so that trends and patterns can be recognised in order to inform future actions and next steps. A planned feedback session can then be used to enable students to respond to common feedback. This can be delivered orally to the class or to a specific group of students to reduce the need for teachers to write repetitive comments on the individual work of each student. This ensures that the quality of feedback is maintained while reducing teachers' workload in relation to written marking and feedback. As with all marking and feedback activities, it is important that a focus on positive praise is maintained. Book sampling may identify common misconceptions, incorrect aspects of subject knowledge or incorrect spelling; however, teachers should seek to draw elements of best practice from the sampling exercise. These could include, for example, the quality of presentation, the complexity and breadth of language used or students' focus on accurate spelling and grammar.

These approaches to marking and feedback can have a significant impact on reducing teachers' workload; however, it is important to identify when these different approaches to feedback may not be suitable. Therefore, it is crucial to remember that written feedback is valuable and has benefits which other forms of feedback cannot offer. For example, it provides a permanent record of interaction that a student can refer back to whereas oral feedback does not. Similarly, whole-class feedback or book sampling may not focus on a complicated or individual need that is specific to an individual student. Thus, teachers must consider their class as a whole while recognising the needs of every individual student. Only then can a decision be made as to the most effective way of securing student progress. Over time, this is likely to involve several approaches being used. Book sampling may be appropriate in one scenario while at another time work may instead require individual and written feedback. To manage workload in relation to marking and feedback, teachers must therefore accept that written feedback is not necessarily the default starting point when beginning to plan any marking and feedback activity. When planning any written feedback, teachers must consider whether another approach to feedback can maintain or increase impact on students' progress while at the same time reducing workload.

CRITICAL QUESTIONS

+ What strategies have you found useful to help you manage your marking workload?

+ Where might you have committed time to written feedback when oral feedback may have had a greater impact?

+ What does the latest Ofsted guidance say about assessment?

DATA MANAGEMENT

Collecting and inputting data can create unnecessary workload for teachers and can have a limited impact on students' progress. Therefore, teachers should understand how their data management activities are going to inform next steps and secure student progress. However, your school is likely to have its own policy in relation to data management and it is important that you adhere to the school's expectations. This policy is likely to outline expectations in relation to the frequency of data input and collection and types of assessment that can be used to inform data collection.

In 2016, the government published the results of its independent report on eliminating unnecessary workload associated with data management. The principles of this report stated that all data management activities should be purposeful, precise and proportionate (DfE, 2016b). Although teachers may have little autonomy and flexibility in relation to their school's data management policy, there are many strategies a teacher can draw on to ensure that their data management is manageable and impactful.

To manage workload, teachers should be ruthless and ask themselves why the data are needed prior to any collection or analysis. If there is no rationale linked to supporting students' progress then the data should not be collected or analysed. However, teachers must align their data management practices with the requirements of school policy. Teachers should streamline their data management by eliminating any duplication and identifying how data can be used more than once. They must also be prepared to stop their data collection and analysis activities and not assume that they should continue simply because they have always taken place previously. Teachers must also be aware of their own workload and consider how long data collection activities will take and whether such time would be better spent on other aspects of professional practice.

Recent regulatory changes – including the removal of levels and Ofsted's decision to no longer examine internal tracking and performance data – should support teachers' workload and it is important that teachers realise and accept that there is no longer an obligation to create elaborate tracking systems and approaches.

When teachers go ahead with data collection and analysis activities, there are several questions to consider in order to ensure that data management is impactful. These include the following.

+ Is the purpose of the data collection and analysis clear? Is there a clear link to students' progress?

+ Are you collecting and analysing data in the most efficient way? Is this work that students could assess themselves? Can you use online software to assess multiple-choice questions automatically?

+ Is the data that you are collecting reliable and valid? Does it actually give you information about progress or attainment?

These questions should allow teachers to challenge themselves and question their current practice within the requirements of school policy. Doing so enables teachers to ensure that data management activities are meaningful and will support improvements in teaching and learning. Although teachers and schools will reach different judgements about the data management activities that are and are not appropriate to their school, subject and age-phase, it is hoped that our discussion will inform adaptations to current practice and support teacher workload.

CRITICAL QUESTIONS

+ What strategies have you found useful to help you manage student progress and achievement data more efficiently?

+ How do you use data on student achievement to inform your planning and teaching?

+ What are the advantages and disadvantages of being 'data rich'?

Recent research by the National Education Union demonstrates the views of more than 8000 teachers in relation to their workload and work–life balance. In summary, the research found that:

- 84 per cent of teachers surveyed said that workload was manageable only sometimes or never;
- 81 per cent of teachers surveyed had considered leaving teaching as a result of workload;
- 34 per cent of teachers surveyed said they can never achieve a good balance between their work and private life.

(NEU, 2018)

CASE STUDY

Tom is in his second year of teaching at a secondary school and sixth form centre. He is the only subject specialist at his school and is responsible for teaching his subject at Key Stage 3, GCSE and A level. During Tom's training year, his mentor shared curriculum and planning resources and Tom was able to use these to support his planning in the first year of his teaching. In his second year of teaching, Tom needed to update and adapt his GCSE and A level resources following specification reform. He also required several new resources for topics that had not been covered by previous specifications. Tom became concerned about his ability and capacity to update existing resources while also needing to create new resources and there were no other subject specialists. Tom created a social media group and asked subject teachers from his local schools to join. The social media group allowed Tom to discuss his planning and collaborate with subject specialists in his local area. Different teachers took responsibility for individual topics and units, and these were then shared through an online file-sharing website. This supported all group members and enabled Tom to manage his workload in relation to lesson planning.

CASE STUDY

Saleema is a primary school teacher and has recently started using an online assessment tool to support her data collection and analysis. The software is able to mark multiple-choice questions and a range of closed questions. These marks are then automatically displayed in a downloadable document that shows performance for each assessment question for the group of students. This allows Saleema to easily identify areas of common strengths and areas for development. The assessment tool has allowed her to reduce the time taken to mark specific assessment questions while maintaining the accuracy and reliability of assessment data. This reduces her workload and ensures that she is able to dedicate sufficient time to the assessment of answers that cannot be marked automatically.

Research by the Department for Education asked teachers to share their experiences, ideas and solutions in relation to unnecessary and unproductive workload. A total of 899 schools were invited to participate in the research and 245 agreed to take part. At least one survey response was received from 218 of these schools, and in total more than 3,000 teachers contributed. In summary, the research found that:

- the average total, self-reported working hours for classroom teachers and middle leaders was 54.4 hours;

- primary classroom teachers and middle leaders self-reported higher total working hours than secondary classroom teachers;

- nearly 33 per cent of part-time teachers reported that 40 per cent of their total hours were worked outside of school hours compared to almost 25 per cent of full-time teachers;

- primary teachers with less than six years' experience reported working a total of 18.8 hours per week outside of school hours, which was two hours more than their experienced primary colleagues and an hour and a half more than secondary teachers with the same level of experience.

(DfE, 2017a)

The problem of teacher stress is pervasive. It is evident across all sectors of education and across countries (Gray et al, 2017) and results in burnout and lower job satisfaction. Teachers are consistently reported to experience an increased risk of developing mental ill-health (Stansfeld et al, 2011; Kidger et al, 2016).

SUMMARY

This chapter has explored some of the challenges you may experience in relation to your own workload. It has drawn on recent research to support you in understanding how teacher workload can impact positive mental health. The chapter has also outlined and explained a range of additional factors known to impact teacher well-being, satisfaction and mental health. A range of practical strategies have been provided to enable you to address and overcome some of the common challenges experienced by teachers in relation to planning, assessment and data management.

CHECKLIST

This chapter has addressed:

✓ some of the factors contributing to teachers disliking their jobs and to teachers' poor mental health;

✓ a range of practical strategies that you can use to support your own workload in relation to planning, assessment and data management.

FURTHER READING

Christodoulou, D (2017) *Making Good Progress? The Future of Assessment for Learning*. Oxford: Oxford University Press.

Spendlove, D (2015) *100 Ideas for Secondary Teachers: Assessment for Learning*. London: Bloomsbury.

✚ CHAPTER 4

DEVELOPING RESILIENCE

PROFESSIONAL LINKS

This chapter addresses the following:

University of Nottingham (2011) *Beyond Survival: Teachers and Resilience*. Nottingham: University of Nottingham.

CHAPTER OBJECTIVES

By the end of this chapter you will understand:

+ the concept of teacher resilience;
+ the factors that shape teacher resilience;
+ strategies to support teacher resilience.

INTRODUCTION

This chapter introduces resilience as a fluid and multi-dimensional concept. It considers definitions of resilience and in doing so attempts to apply these to teaching. Additionally, the chapter demonstrates why resilience is important in teaching. Greenfield's (2015) model of teacher resilience is then considered in order to illustrate a range of factors which shape and inform teacher resilience. The chapter then draws on research to provide and discuss a number of common coping strategies that teachers use to stay resilient.

WHAT IS RESILIENCE?

Resilience is multi-dimensional and context specific. Teachers can demonstrate varying levels of resilience in the different contexts that they inhabit and therefore it is better to view resilience as a dynamic rather than static construct. Some define resilience in terms of physical continuation in the role (Hong, 2012) or 'staying power', while others view resilience more in terms of the ability to sustain motivation, commitment and, therefore, effectiveness in the profession (Day, 2008). There is an increasing tendency to think of resilience as the ability to *'thrive rather than just survive'* (Beltman et al, 2011, p 186).

Although some academics continue to define resilience as a personal quality (Brunetti, 2006), others have raised concerns that 'within-person' perspectives on resilience fail to recognise systemic influences that shape teacher resilience. Teacher resilience can be influenced by educational policy, school climate and access to external networks of support. Therefore, 'within-person' perspectives fail to recognise that the interaction between individual, relational and contextual or organisational factors affect resilience (Greenfield, 2015).

WHY IS RESILIENCE IMPORTANT?

Teaching is an increasingly demanding job which requires significant levels of resilience. Most teachers will experience a range of professional challenges which they need to be resilient to. These might include:

+ dealing with abusive parents and parental complaints;

+ managing challenging behaviour from students;

+ coping with 'difficult' colleagues;

+ working with unsupportive school leaders;

+ surviving school inspections;

+ working within a challenging policy climate;

+ coping with threats of redundancy;

+ working within limited school budgets;

+ working in toxic school cultures;

+ coping with personal challenges.

This is not an exhaustive list but, nevertheless, it illustrates clearly that resilience is necessary to address some of these challenges. Most teachers become increasingly more resilient with greater experience. They somehow manage to cope in even the most challenging situations. For early career teachers, their confidence can easily be knocked through negative interactions with others. The good news for teachers is that resilience is not a fixed characteristic. It can be developed and nurtured, and a range of strategies to foster resilience are suggested later in this chapter.

WHAT FACTORS INFLUENCE TEACHER RESILIENCE?

Teacher resilience is often understood as a relative and dynamic quality (Day and Gu, 2007) which is influenced by a combination of factors, some of which are external to the individual. Greenfield's (2015) model of teacher resilience is useful because it identifies a range of factors which shape teacher resilience. The model is presented below, in Figure 4.1.

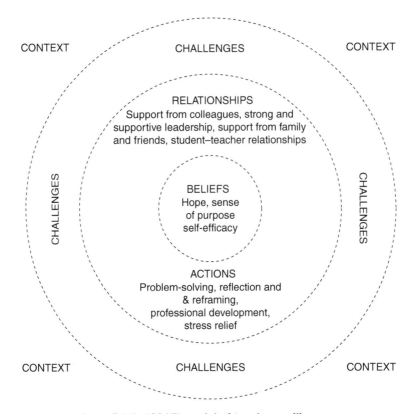

Figure 4.1 Greenfield's (2015) model of teacher resilience.

+ Beliefs. Teachers' beliefs about themselves and their role can
  significantly influence their resilience. Teachers with high levels
  of self-efficacy (beliefs that teachers hold about their capabilities)
  are more likely to develop resilient qualities (Gu and Day, 2013).
  According to Greenfield (2015), when teachers have a sense of
  purpose and hope they tend to be more resilient than teachers who
  lack these.

+ Relationships. Social connectivity with others influences resilience.
  According to Greenfield (2015), teachers with strong connections
  with colleagues, leaders, students, friends and family are more
  likely to be resilient because these connections provide them
  with access to support networks. Having limited or no social
  connections can impact detrimentally on teacher resilience in some
  cases but not necessarily in all cases.

+ Actions. According to Greenfield (2015), the actions that teachers
  adopt can influence their resilience. For example, if teachers

seek help from others, solve problems, engage in rejuvenation and renewal and skilfully manage difficult relationships, this can increase their resilience.

+ Challenges. The challenges that teachers experience may be personal or professional and these can influence their resilience. For example, Glazzard and Rose (2019) found that teachers' experiences of domestic violence and parental illness can have a detrimental effect on their resilience and overall well-being. The ability to cope with personal challenges can also be diminished if teachers possess poor self-efficacy. In addition, lack of opportunities to gain support from others can also influence teachers' abilities to cope with challenges and this can impact detrimentally on their resilience. Thus, the factors identified in Greenfield (2015) are interrelated. Professional challenges, including the breakdown of relationships in school, changes to school leadership teams, the introduction of new policies and negative outcomes in school inspections, can influence teacher resilience.

+ Context. The personal and professional contexts which shape teachers' lives can influence their resilience (Greenfield, 2015). The broader educational context (for example, the focus on raising educational attainment) can influence teachers' self-efficacy, their relationships with others and the challenges they experience in their own professional context. Changes in teachers' personal circumstances (divorce, separation, family or personal illness) can also influence their resilience.

CRITICAL QUESTIONS

+ What are the strengths and limitations of this model?

+ Can you identify any elements which are missing from the model?

+ To what extent might a focus on 'actions' in Greenfield's model place the onus on the individual teacher, thus detracting from the systemic forces which impact detrimentally on resilience?

Recent research by the National Education Union (2017) found that over 80 per cent of teachers had considered leaving the profession during the past year because of workload.

Teachers cited the following reasons as the cause of unsustainable workload demands.

- 74 per cent said pressure to increase student scores and grades.

- 52 per cent said changes to curriculum, assessment and exams.

- 46 per cent said Ofsted, mock inspections and other inspections.

- 41 per cent said lack of money and resources in the school.

- 33 per cent said demands from school leaders and governors.

- 33 per cent said reduction of support staff.

(NEU, 2017)

STRATEGIES TO SUPPORT TEACHER RESILIENCE

Research has found a number of common coping strategies that teachers use to stay resilient. Individual strategies include:

+ *being organised;*

+ *limiting the amount of work they do at home;*

+ *protecting time for hobbies;*

+ *talking to family and friends;*

+ *choosing to work reduced hours;*

+ *participating in physical activity.*

(Glazzard and Rose, 2019)

School-level strategies include:

+ *developing a staff well-being policy;*

+ *introducing staff buddy systems for informal and confidential support;*

+ *including a well-being target in staff performance management arrangements;*

+ *developing whole-school policies to reduce teacher workload;*

+ *introducing phased returns and flexible working arrangements.*

(Glazzard and Rose, 2019)

CRITICAL QUESTIONS

+ What strategies do you employ to be resilient?

+ What factors influence your own resilience as a teacher in your own professional and personal contexts?

CASE STUDY

Reuben is a middle leader and has been teaching in a secondary school for four years. In the third year of his career, Reuben was appointed to his middle leadership position and became responsible for a team of seven teaching staff within his subject area. During the same academic year, he experienced significant challenges in his personal life, and he began to find these pressures difficult to manage alongside his new leadership role. As an inexperienced leader and a teacher with only four years of experience, he felt that he had not yet developed sufficient resilience to cope with these challenges and pressures without seeking additional support. He had recognised that he felt he could not cope and decided to speak to his employer rather than 'plough on' as if everything was fine. The employer offered confidential non-judgemental advice and made Reuben aware of the counselling and support services available both through the school and teaching union. Reuben's employer provided a flexible working agreement which allowed him to focus on the challenges he was experiencing in his personal life. Upon his return to work, a senior colleague was given some of Reuben's responsibilities to ensure that his phased return to work was manageable and that the quality of his teaching and leadership was not compromised.

RECOGNISING WHEN YOU ARE NOT COPING

It is important to listen to warning signs that your body communicates to you when you are not coping. Signs could include feeling stressed, breathlessness, panic attacks, low mood, self-imposed isolation, headaches, insomnia and changes in diet and physical appearance. This is not an exhaustive list and the signs will vary between individuals. The important thing is to acknowledge that you are not coping and to seek help from others that you trust as soon as possible before the problem escalates. It is important not to 'plough on' as if everything is fine. Do not be afraid to take advice from your doctor and do not feel afraid or guilty about taking time off work if you need this to help you recover. Your employer has a duty of care to you and therefore must give priority to your well-being. Talk to people who will listen to you without judging you.

CRITICAL QUESTIONS

+ What are the warning signs that someone is not coping?

+ If you notice that a colleague is not coping, what might you do next?

Teachers sometimes continue to work even if they are ill. They try to be resilient because they may be worried about letting students and colleagues down and they may be worried about how their absence from school might be perceived by senior leaders. However, research demonstrates that teachers who demonstrate 'presenteeism' find it more difficult to manage their classrooms effectively (Jennings and Greenberg, 2009) and are less likely to develop positive classroom and behaviour management strategies (Harding et al, 2019). Presenteeism is evident when teachers with poor well-being and mental health continue to work. The quality of their work is reduced, and this affects the quality of their relationships with their students (Jennings and Greenberg, 2009), student well-being (Harding et al, 2019) and overall teacher performance (Beck et al, 2011; Jain et al, 2013).

SEEKING HELP

If you recognise that you need help, there are various ways of accessing help. You might be able to gain sufficient support from colleagues, friends, partners or other members of your family. Some schools and local authorities offer a free confidential counselling service to staff. You might not require this but it is important to know that it is available if you need it. If you are a member of a teaching union and you feel that work-related stress has impacted detrimentally on your well-being and resilience, you can contact your school representative or regional officer for confidential advice. Additionally, you can also access support from the Education Support Partnership (www.educationsupportpartnership.org.uk)

CRITICAL QUESTIONS

+ What are the barriers to seeking help for teachers?

+ How might you encourage a colleague to seek help?

MAINTAINING YOUR MORAL PURPOSE

Greenfield's (2015) model identifies the importance of having a sense of purpose and links this to teacher resilience. When you experience difficult times in your teaching career, try to remember why you are a teacher. Most teachers are intrinsically motivated to make a positive difference to their students. Sometimes it is easy to lose sight of this, especially when you become embroiled in internal politics within the school. Hold on to your core motivations during these times and remember the positive impact that you are having on young people. Teaching is a deeply rewarding but challenging profession. However, the rewards outweigh the challenges and remembering this will help you during challenging times.

CRITICAL QUESTIONS

+ What drives you in your career?

+ How would you rate your own teacher efficacy and how does this affect your resilience?

Recent research by the Education Support Partnership examined the support that was accessed by education professionals who have experienced mental health issues. The research, published in the Teacher Wellbeing Index (2018), also surveyed teachers' perceptions of the types of support available. Key statistics demonstrate the following:

- In 2017, 24 per cent of education professionals who experienced mental health issues at work did not speak to anybody about it.

- In 2018, 26 per cent of education professionals who experienced mental health issues at work did not speak to anybody about it.

- In 2017 and 2018, 36 per cent of education professionals those who did not speak to anybody about their mental health issues at work stated that this was because they would see it as a sign of weakness.

- In 2017 and 2018, 17 per cent of those who did not speak to anybody about their mental health issues at work stated that this was because they were worried about losing their job.

- In 2017, of those who did speak to someone at work or outside work, 54 per cent felt that the discussion gave them perspective and helped them realise they were not alone.

- In 2018, of those who did speak to someone at work or outside work, 48 per cent felt that the discussion gave them perspective and helped them realise they were not alone.

- In 2017, 4 per cent of those surveyed reported having access to resilience, energy or stress management classes or programmes.

- In 2018, 5 per cent of those surveyed reported having access to resilience, energy or stress management classes or programmes.

(ESP, 2018)

CASE STUDY

Jamila was in her second year of teaching and worked in a small department where there were no other teaching staff with the same subject specialism. She completed her first year of teaching in a different school. Her line manager, Tom, had been absent for several months and Jamila had been dealing with parental complaints on his behalf. Jamila had also been setting cover for Tom's lessons and she continued to try and plan all of her own lessons from scratch as there were no departmental resources. Jamila became increasingly anxious about her ability to cope and began to have sleepless nights. She decided not to share her concerns with school leaders as she felt they were unsupportive and judgemental. She also felt that there was no need to talk to anyone about her concerns as she had realised that she could work for several hours every evening and at weekends to keep up with the demands placed on her.

Jamila was sleeping for approximately three hours per night. She felt that she was being resilient to the challenges she was experiencing as her students and colleagues were not being let down by her absence or reduced output. She also did not need to worry about senior leaders being judgemental as they did not know about her anxiety and stress. However, Jamila's attempts to 'plough on' became counter-productive. Colleagues became concerned about Jamila as she began to make regular mistakes and errors. Colleagues also noticed that Jamila had started to 'snap' at her students. Jamila had not realised that she was beginning to experience 'presenteeism'. Eventually, her anxiety and stress became too serious to manage, resulting in long-term absence.

Jamila eventually returned to work with the support of a counsellor and her teaching union. She now runs a staff well-being group and uses this forum to share her story and encourage colleagues to seek help from others that they trust, as soon as possible, to avoid problems escalating. She also leads discussions in relation to common coping strategies and now recognises and promotes the importance of communicating with others and seeking support.

Doney (2012) found the relational support system was 'the most frequently used protective factor to counteract stressors' (p 656). In addition, Huisman et al (2010) found that teachers cited significant adult relationships as their primary source of support. The link between relationships and resilience has been highlighted in a range of studies (Le Cornu, 2009, 2013; Papatraianou and Le Cornu, 2014). Gu and Day (2013) highlight how mutually appreciative relationships with school leaders can increase teacher efficacy. Huisman et al (2010) highlight the important role that mentors can play in increasing hope, which influences resilience (Greenfield, 2015). Research has found that positive relationships with students can contribute towards teachers' self-efficacy (Doney, 2012), which plays a critical role in enhancing resilience (Greenfield, 2015).

SUMMARY

This chapter has explored resilience as a fluid and multi-dimensional concept. It has considered definitions of resilience and in doing so has attempted to apply these to teaching. The chapter has demonstrated why resilience is important in teaching and Greenfield's (2015) model of teacher resilience has been used to illustrate a range of factors which shape and inform teacher resilience. Research has also been considered to provide and discuss a number of common coping strategies that teachers use to stay resilient.

CHECKLIST

This chapter has addressed:

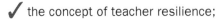

✓ the concept of teacher resilience;

✓ the factors that shape teacher resilience;

✓ strategies to support teacher resilience.

FURTHER READING

Busch, B and Watson, E (2019) *The Science of Learning: 77 Studies That Every Teacher Needs to Know*. Abingdon: Routledge.

Simister, C (2017) *Character, Grit and Resilience Pocketbook*. Alresford: Teachers' Pocketbooks.

✛ CHAPTER 5

MANAGING BEHAVIOUR

PROFESSIONAL LINKS

This chapter addresses the following:

The Teachers' Standards state that teachers must:

⊘ have clear rules and routines for behaviour in classrooms, and take responsibility for promoting good and courteous behaviour both in classrooms and around the school, in accordance with the school's behaviour policy;

⊘ have high expectations of behaviour and establish a framework for discipline with a range of strategies, using praise, sanctions and rewards consistently and fairly.

CHAPTER OBJECTIVES

By the end of this chapter you will understand:

+ the link between student behaviour and teacher mental health;

+ strategies for managing students' behaviour.

INTRODUCTION

This chapter outlines how to manage students' behaviour in lessons and how to promote good behaviour for learning. Many teachers have sleepless nights where they worry about students' behaviour. It is easy to interpret negative behaviour as a personal response to you. However, this is rarely the case. Sadly, some young people have experienced adverse childhood experiences and these may affect their behaviour in school. Some may have developed a poor sense of self and this can detrimentally impact on their behaviour. Although poor behaviour is draining, it is important that you try to understand its root causes. Sanctions provide a 'quick fix' but they do not address the causes. This chapter outlines some important strategies that will support you in managing students' behaviour.

CRITICAL QUESTIONS

+ Reflect on your own style for managing students' behaviour. What are your preferred approaches and why do you like them?

+ Reflect on approaches that you have observed that have been effective and less effective. What factors influenced the effectiveness of these approaches?

DEVELOPING POSITIVE RELATIONSHIPS

Establishing positive relationships with students is the starting point to support you in developing good behaviour management. While this will not necessarily guarantee good behaviour, it will reduce the likelihood of negative behaviour occurring. Students generally do not learn from teachers that they do not like. Your students need to know that:

+ you care for them as people as well as caring for their learning;

+ you understand them;

+ you believe in them;

+ you will forgive them when they get things wrong.

Although you will need to establish clear behavioural expectations in every lesson, students generally enjoy lessons if they like the teacher. Students tend not to like teachers who shout and it is often true that a noisy teacher produces a noisy class. Try not to shout unless absolutely necessary and deal with issues firmly but calmly. It is easier to start firm and then subsequently relax with a class. All students will test you at first, so a 'no-nonsense' approach is best adopted. You should find that when students are clear about your behavioural expectations, you will then be able to relax with them and demonstrate a sense of humour as time progresses. The following list includes simple and effective ways of establishing relationships with new classes.

+ Learn the names of all students very quickly; a seating plan will help with this.

+ Smile.

+ Try to get to know your students, including their interests outside of school.

+ Thank them for their contributions in class.

+ Acknowledge the effort they make with their work.

+ Create a 'can-do' culture so that students start to believe in their abilities.

+ Apologise to students if you make a mistake.

+ Tell them a little about yourself.

+ Be enthusiastic about your teaching; if you are excited, it will be infectious.

+ Use eye contact.

+ Use students' names in class.

RULES AND ROUTINES

Establishing clear expectations for students' behaviour is critical and it is important that you follow the whole-school policy in relation to rules and routines. Simple strategies such as greeting the students as they enter the classroom set the correct tone for the rest of the lesson. Displaying a task on the board for them to do as soon as they sit down ensures that there is no wasted learning time and this will minimise disruption. Establish clear expectations about punctuality to lessons and implement sanctions if students turn up to lessons late. Read the school behaviour policy and ensure that you are familiar with the rules and routines of the school. If these are consistently applied by all teachers, students clearly understand what is expected of them. Establish basic expectations. These include the following.

+ When you talk, they must listen.

+ Mobile phones must be turned off and kept in their bags.

+ Insist that they listen carefully when other students are answering questions or making other contributions to the lessons.

+ Insist that they value everyone's contribution.

+ Establish a zero-tolerance policy on use of bad language in class and implement sanctions where necessary.

+ Develop clear rules on whether movement around the classroom is permitted.

+ Develop clear routines and expectations at the end of lessons, for example, tidying away, pushing chairs under, picking things up from the floor, and explain clearly to students what they should do if you are still talking and the bell goes.

+ Develop rules for classroom talk – when is it allowed and when is it not?

+ Develop clear rules for tasks – be clear about whether students should be working individually or whether they are allowed to collaborate.

+ Ensure that students do not eat food in lessons or chew gum.

+ Not permitting the wearing of hats or coats in the classroom.

+ Not permitting disrespect of school property, for example, by adding graffiti onto their exercise books.

These are examples of classroom rules but your school behaviour policy will guide you on the expectations. If you notice low-level disruption, 'nip this in the bud' immediately by challenging it. Ignoring it creates a culture of low expectations and often the problem will grow into a bigger problem if it is unchallenged.

CRITICAL QUESTIONS

+ Do you agree or disagree with the rules listed above? Explain your response.

+ Are there any other rules which should be included in this list?

PRAISE AND REWARDS

Take every opportunity to praise good behaviour and good effort. Assign rewards in line with the school policy. Although students generally enjoy receiving praise and rewards, and their use results in other students modifying their behaviour, there are some issues that you need to take into consideration.

+ The over-use of praise can result in a culture of low expectations, particularly when praise is given when it is not really deserved.

+ It can result in students working hard only because they want a reward; this promotes extrinsic motivation rather than intrinsic motivation.

+ Rewards and praise tend to be assigned to students who do not demonstrate consistently good behaviour; when they suddenly modify their behaviour, they tend to receive praise or rewards.

+ Some students never receive rewards or praise; these tend to be students who work hard and behave well consistently.

CRITICAL QUESTIONS

+ What are your views on the use of praise and rewards?

+ How can teachers promote intrinsic rather than extrinsic motivation?

USING SANCTIONS

Sanctions should be applied either when students' attitudes to learning are not good or when they demonstrate inappropriate behaviour. You must implement sanctions in line with school policy during your lessons and sanctions should be proportionate to the incident that warranted their use.

CRITICAL QUESTIONS

+ What are your views on the use of isolation?

+ What are the advantages and disadvantages of using sanctions?

Through operant conditioning, a child makes an association between a particular behaviour and a consequence (Skinner, 1938). The underlying principle is that positive reinforcement of good behaviour strengthens that behaviour. In addition, negative reinforcement (often incorrectly associated with punishment) is the removal of an adverse experience to avoid a negative outcome. Negative reinforcement strengthens the desired behaviour.

CLASSROOM MANAGEMENT

One effective strategy for developing good classroom management is to implement a seating plan. This enables you to learn students' names quickly and to separate students who are likely to disrupt each other. Follow the school policies on whether students are allowed to leave their seats during lessons and on toilet use during lessons. Make sure that your expectations are clear from the moment they enter the room. Giving them a task to do immediately is one way of settling them down and focusing them on learning.

PROMOTING POSITIVE LEARNING BEHAVIOUR

In recent years, there has been a move away from the term 'behaviour management' to 'behaviour for learning', despite the former term being adopted in the Teachers' Standards. Students demonstrate good behaviour for learning when they are:

+ listening;

+ collaborating;

+ asking questions;

+ challenging other people's opinions about subject content;

+ persevering when they find something difficult;

+ managing distractions;

+ making connections between different aspects of learning;

+ noticing;

+ being independent;

+ using tools for learning when they become 'stuck' rather than depending on a teacher.

Some students find it difficult to participate in lessons. They do not ask questions and they tend to be passive. Quiet, passive and compliant behaviour is not good learning behaviour. You need to encourage your students to ask questions, to affirm other people's responses or to challenge them to persevere when they are working on a really difficult problem. Effective learners manage their distractions well. If there is disruption taking place, or if someone walks into the room to talk to you, effective learners manage these distractions well and continue on their task. Some students waste valuable learning time when they become 'stuck' in their learning. This stops them from making progress in the lesson. Through teaching the students a four-step process, you can offer them a framework to guide their response when this happens. When students become 'stuck' you can encourage them to:

+ think;

+ talk to a peer;

+ use tools for learning (resources to help them with their learning);

+ talk to a teacher.

The 'four t's' approach ensures that the last thing they do if they become stuck is to ask a teacher. When you see students demonstrating good learning behaviours, you should provide positive descriptive praise, for example: *'I liked the way you persevered with that task, Sam'*; *'I saw some really great collaboration in that group'*.

The Teacher Wellbeing Index is research published by the Education Support Partnership. In 2018, the research demonstrated that an overwhelming majority of the UK's education professionals suffered physical and mental health issues as a result of their jobs (ESP, 2018). One aspect of the research surveyed education professionals who had experienced symptoms (behavioural, physical or psychological) due to work or where work was a contributing factor. The results of the survey included:

- students' behaviour being a work issue: 43 per cent of the education professionals surveyed in 2018 attributed their symptoms to this;

- students' behaviour being a work issue: 34 per cent of the education professionals surveyed in 2017 attributed their symptoms to this;

- 60 per cent of staff who felt threatened reporting that such threats had come from students.

(ESP, 2018)

CASE STUDY

Mario, an NQT, was recently signed off by his GP on the grounds of stress and anxiety. Mario was given three months of sick leave after having a breakdown at work. Prior to his teacher training and subsequent employment as an NQT, he had never experienced mental ill-health. Poor student behaviour and a lack of support from senior leaders in the school left him feeling undermined and bullied, which caused stress and anxiety. Mario reported being sick prior to work and experiencing nightmares several times per week. He had considered leaving the school or the profession many times but felt a professional commitment to his students and their education. His refusal to leave the school had eventually resulted in his mental ill-health and subsequent absence from work. He had never confronted the leadership team as he feared dismissal.

While on long-term absence, Mario decided to leave the school and subsequently secured a teaching post elsewhere. In his new school, he felt supported by colleagues and leaders. There was a culture of high expectation in which all staff were empowered and supported to challenge poor behaviour. Mario's confidence grew. He no longer feared going to work. In his current role, he now works with trainees on teacher training programmes and delivers development sessions on behaviour and engagement to colleagues from across the school. He continues to share his story to demonstrate the importance of working in the right school with the right approach to staff well-being, culture and student behaviour.

SOLUTION-FOCUSED APPROACHES

Solution-focused conversations are positive conversations that you might have with a student. The aim is to develop a positive sense of self and to set small, achievable goals. This approach is used by many psychologists and it is based on Carl Roger's concept of *unconditional positive regard*. Many students who demonstrate poor behaviour are locked in a negative cycle. They are reprimanded and sanctions are imposed on them. Although this approach is not meant to replace the use of sanctions, it can provide a contrasting approach at a different time when the focus shifts from negative conversations to positive conversations. The conversation is carried out through a series of questions which support the student to reflect on their social and emotional development. The student is positioned as the expert, rather than the adult. The skill of the adult is to pick up on what the student is saying in the conversation and to use this as a springboard for questioning. Not all elements of the solution-focused approach are identified below but typically sessions will include the following.

+ Problem-free talk: These conversations focus on the individual's strengths. Questions might include: What do you think your friends or parents might say are your strengths? What are you good at? What do you enjoy doing?

+ Acknowledgement: This provides an opportunity for you to acknowledge the student's difficulties but also to compliment them on how they have addressed/are addressing their difficulties.

+ Finding exceptions: This provides an opportunity to ask questions which focus on times when the student has demonstrated positive behaviour. For example, 'Can you describe a time when you felt angry but stayed calm?'

+ Scaling activities: These provide an opportunity for the student to rate themselves and to set goals. A visual or physical rating scale can be used. For example, 'On a scale of 1 to 10 (1 = poor; 10 = brilliant), how would you rate your confidence/motivation/ behaviour/being in control/anxiousness? Why have you chosen this score? What score would you like to reach in a month's time? What will you be doing that might be different by then?'

+ Follow-up sessions: These provide an opportunity to find out what is going well for the student. Questions might include: 'What's going well for you? What have you been pleased with? What has been your greatest achievement since we last met?'

CASE STUDY

Aiysha was an English teacher. A student in one of her classes was particularly disruptive and this was having a detrimental impact on the learning of other students. Aiysha decided to talk to the student to find out what might be causing the problem. The student said that he was 'rubbish' at English because he found the text too difficult. Aiysha told the student that although he found the text difficult now, this did not mean that he would not be able to eventually understand it. Aiysha decided to give the student one specific task to focus on each week relating to the text. This meant that he had read the relevant aspect of the text prior to coming to lessons. Over several weeks, his confidence gradually improved and so too did his behaviour.

In 2018, the Department for Education published statistics in relation to the number and rate of permanent exclusions and the reasons for these. These statistics demonstrated that:

● the overall rate of permanent exclusions had increased from 0.08 per cent of student enrolments in 2015/16 to 0.10 per cent in 2016/17;

● the number of permanent exclusions increased from 6685 to 7720 from 2015/16 to 2016/17;

- the overall rate of fixed period exclusions had increased from 4.29 per cent of student enrolments in 2015/16 to 4.76 per cent in 2016/17;

- the number of fixed period exclusions increased from 339,360 to 381,865 from 2015/16 to 2016/17;

- there were 2755 exclusions for persistent disruptive behaviour in 2016/17, up from 2310 exclusions in 2015/16;

- there were 655 exclusions for verbal assault against an adult in 2016/17, up from 600 exclusions in 2015/16;

- the number of exclusions for verbal assault against a student, sexual misconduct, racist abuse, physical assault against a student, physical assault against an adult, damage and in relation to drugs and alcohol also increased from 2015/16 to 2016/17.

(DfE, 2018c)

In 2016, the Department for Education commissioned a research study to review behaviour management practices in schools. The review drew on evidence from a variety of sources. These included observations, headteacher and expert panels and the use of desk research. The study involved undertaking qualitative research into behaviour management practices used in schools that had been categorised as outstanding by Ofsted, having improved their inspection outcome since their previous Ofsted rating.

The study identified ten themes which emerged from the research undertaken. The research emphasised that these themes under-pinned overall approaches to behaviour management rather than specific strategies. The research acknowledged that any strategies employed had to be tweaked to reflect school, teacher and local population context, and that they must be reviewed, refined and updated through time.

The ten key themes identified were:

+ policies and practice;

+ structures;

+ general behaviour practice;

+ rewards and praise;

+ sanctions;

+ Special Educational Needs and Disabilities (SEND) provision;

+ data;

+ parents and other agencies;

+ culture and ethos;

+ consistency.

Although these findings are drawn from a limited sample size, they demonstrate the importance of balancing positive reinforcement and behavioural modelling with clearly defined processes for tackling and addressing poor behaviour. The findings also highlight the importance of school culture and ethos, led by senior leaders who recognise and understand the school context and its requirements. These approaches are therefore likely to support teacher well-being and it is important that teachers can recognise, inform and challenge the development of institutional policy.

(DfE, 2017b)

SUMMARY

This chapter has explored how to manage students' behaviour in lessons and how to promote good behaviour for learning. We have acknowledged that it is common for many teachers to feel anxious about students' behaviour and that it is important to recognise that negative behaviour is usually not directed at you personally. In some cases, adverse childhood experiences may be affecting students' behaviour and these individuals may have developed a poor sense of self as a result of these experiences. The chapter has explained that it is important that teachers recognise that this can detrimentally impact on student behaviour and that behavioural responses should not be taken personally. Therefore, it is important that you try to understand the root causes of behaviour and ask for support whenever you feel that this would be valuable. However, it is important to recognise that teachers do have an influence on students' behaviour and the chapter has outlined some important strategies that will support you with managing behaviour.

CHECKLIST

This chapter has addressed:

✓ the link between student behaviour and teacher mental health;

✓ strategies for managing students' behaviour.

FURTHER READING

Cowley, S (2014) *Getting the Buggers to Behave*. London: Bloomsbury Publishing.

Porter, L (2014) *Behaviour in Schools: Theory and Practice for Teachers*. Maidenhead: Open University Press.

✛ CHAPTER 6

MANAGING PROFESSIONAL RELATIONSHIPS

PROFESSIONAL LINKS

This chapter addresses the following:

The Teachers' Standards state that teachers must:

- develop effective professional relationships with colleagues, knowing how and when to draw on advice and specialist support;

- take responsibility for improving teaching through appropriate professional development, responding to advice and feedback from colleagues.

CHAPTER OBJECTIVES

By the end of this chapter you will understand:

+ the importance of developing effective relationships with colleagues, senior leaders and governors;

+ ways of overcoming a range of common problems that you may encounter in relation to professional relationships.

INTRODUCTION

This chapter outlines the role of school-based mentors in supporting and assessing trainees. It also emphasises the importance of the trainee and mentor developing an effective relationship and strategies are suggested to support this. Additionally, the chapter provides practical advice on managing relationships with colleagues, senior leaders and governors, and some critical questions are offered to encourage you to reflect on your own professional relationships.

MANAGING RELATIONSHIPS WITH MENTORS DURING YOUR ITT AND NQT PHASES

Developing effective relationships with mentors has been addressed in Chapter 2. School-based mentors play a pivotal role in ITT placements. They play a dual role in that they are required to develop and support trainees, but at the same time they are also responsible for assessing trainees. When relationships break down between trainees and mentors, it can have a serious impact on the placement and, in the worst-case scenario, it can lead to placements being terminated.

Trainees therefore need to invest time into developing effective relationships with their mentors. Simple strategies for doing this include:

+ being enthusiastic and conscientious;

+ demonstrating hard work, effort and commitment;

+ listening to and acting on mentor advice;

+ reflecting on own practice;

+ demonstrating a high standard of professionalism;

+ being respectful of the mentor's time and efforts.

This is not an exhaustive list but it does illustrate the importance of adopting a highly professional approach when working in schools. If relationships are breaking down, it is best to address this immediately by talking to your mentor or by discussing it with a representative from your ITT provider.

Research by Glazzard and Coverdale (2018) demonstrates that the NQTs in their study emphasised the importance of having an effective mentor. The research was a small-scale case study of eight participants who were in the first year of teaching in the primary phase (5–11). The NQTs characterised an effective mentor as someone who was supportive and able to provide constructive feedback on their teaching. The participants indicated that they valued formal and informal support from their mentor and they recognised the importance of establishing a good relationship. Glazzard and Coverdale's (2018) research also demonstrates that NQTs find it useful to have access to a network of support from other people including teaching assistants, parents and other teachers in the school. Therefore, it is important that mentors create and highlight opportunities for trainees and NQTs to develop and access these networks. This is particularly crucial when such colleagues are relatively new to a placement or school context and may find it difficult to access these support networks without the additional support and guidance of their mentor. Effective mentoring is pivotal to the success of an induction year or training placement. It is therefore crucial that the trainee and mentor work together to develop their relationship throughout their time together.

Research by Sue Griffiths (2011) on the experiences of trainee teachers with dyslexia demonstrates how they felt unsupported in schools by their mentors and were often subjected to criticism. She states:

> Within the teaching profession, a paradoxical situation exists where trainees and teachers with dyslexia can feel being dyslexic confers advantages and offers unique insights into difficulties experienced by the children they are teaching, yet are undervalued, unsupported and regarded... as being detrimental to the profession.

(Griffiths, 2011, p 60)

Griffiths (2011) found that mentors felt that they had a duty to act as gatekeepers to the profession through not allowing unsuitable entrants into it, yet at the same time they knew that they have a legal duty to make reasonable adjustments to placements to ensure that trainee teachers with dyslexia had equality of opportunity. However, there was often a lack of a pro-active approach towards meeting the needs of these trainees, resulting in them feeling undervalued, unsupported and damaged by the placement.

CASE STUDY

Nash began his teacher training in September and began his school-based training in October. He was anxious about the training placement and was keen to develop an effective relationship with his mentor. Nash arranged to meet his mentor once per week and asked how he could contribute to the relationship. He took an active approach and arranged to shadow his mentor regularly. After each shadowing session, he prepared three questions that related to his mentor's approach to teaching. He shared these questions with his mentor in advance of the mentor meeting to allow the mentor time to consider and prepare responses. Nash was also pro-active in preparing and sharing the weekly agenda and always sent this in advance of the deadline. Nash was honest with his mentor about his feelings and emotions and always sought and responded to advice thoughtfully and professionally. Nash also asked his mentor to recommend other teachers to work with and shadow and called on these colleagues as part of his extended support network. Throughout the placement, Nash was able to build an effective relationship with his mentor. He completed his placement successfully and believes that his approach to collaboration, communication and commitment underpinned this success.

CRITICAL QUESTIONS

+ What are the attributes of a good ITT mentor?
+ What factors can cause relationships between trainee teachers and their mentors to break down?

MANAGING RELATIONSHIPS WITH OTHER COLLEAGUES IN SCHOOL

Developing good relationships with colleagues in school is critical for your well-being as a teacher. Schools are social places and teachers thrive when there is a sense of collegiality and mutual support. Other colleagues in school can also provide you with valuable support networks if you start to experience challenges in either your personal life or professional life. Colleagues can help by providing you with a friendly listening ear, taking on some of your workload and by suggesting solutions to your problems.

At the same time, you will encounter colleagues who do the exact opposite. They create stress for you, are critical of your teaching, try to compete with you and attempt to undermine you. These colleagues are a drain on your energy and over time their negativity can result in you developing poor mental health. The best thing that you can do in these circumstances is to distance yourself from people like this. Try to surround yourself with people who radiate positivity and do your best to distance yourself from colleagues who may simply be jealous of your own success.

The situation is trickier to deal with if you are line managed by a colleague who consistently tries to undermine you. In this situation it is important to document what is happening. Keep a diary of incidents which occur. Include dates and times and an outline of each incident which occurs. You may need to present the diary as evidence if you decide to take out a grievance against a colleague on the grounds of bullying or harassment. If you suspect that you are being victimised, it is better to raise the issue directly with the colleague who is mistreating you. If you feel uncomfortable going into meetings alone with this colleague, you have a right to take a colleague into the meeting with you for mutual support. Reflect on the reasons why they might be treating you like this and if necessary contact your teaching union for confidential advice.

CRITICAL QUESTIONS

+ What are the factors that can result in a teacher being harassed or bullied?

+ Have you ever been treated like this in the workplace? If so, how have you dealt with it in the past?

+ What are the attributes of good colleagues who you align yourself with?

+ What are the warning signs that you might be experiencing bullying, harassment or discrimination?

ESTABLISHING EFFECTIVE RELATIONSHIPS WITH SENIOR LEADERS

Senior leaders in school are in a position of power and consequently can potentially significantly influence the quality of your working life and your career. Investing time in developing effective and positive relationships with senior leaders is a good use of your time and it will make your life easier in the long run.

However, holding a position of power does not give anyone a right to bully other colleagues. This constitutes a serious abuse of power and it does not create positive school cultures which are essential for mentally healthy schools. The revised Ofsted framework (Ofsted, 2019) provides inspectors with the power to investigate and challenge workplace bullying, and this is a positive development. However, many teachers are too frightened to report workplace bullying because they are scared of damaging their own professional reputation and worried about the implications for their own careers. It is important that you research members of a school's leadership team when applying for jobs. Professional bullies will often hold reputations locally and other teachers or heads may be aware of their tactics. It is better to avoid working with people like this if at all possible because you will likely end up working within a toxic school environment.

When accepting employment in a school, it is important to develop effective working relationships with senior leaders. Examples include:

+ working hard;

+ meeting deadlines;

+ not being confrontational;

+ listening to and acting on constructive advice;

+ keeping senior leaders informed about your practice;

+ taking on reasonable additional responsibilities in school when asked;

+ putting students first;

+ demonstrating the highest level of professionalism.

However, in your efforts to please people, it is important that you do not become the 'go to' person for tasks which leaders need to allocate. Enthusiastic teachers who always agree to additional responsibilities can easily become overwhelmed as they take on more and more additional commitments. This can result in them becoming stressed and it can impact detrimentally on your mental health, the quality of your relationships and your teaching.

In March 2018, the Department for Education published a report on its research into the factors affecting teacher retention. The research consisted of a survey being sent to former teachers and was disseminated through the *TES* and subject associations. The survey gave a range of reasons for leaving teaching and asked former teachers about their current employment status. The purpose of the research was to further explore the reasons why teachers leave the profession and to understand what would encourage them to remain in or return to the profession. In summary, the research demonstrated that:

- 85 per cent of respondents cited a lack of support from leadership as one of the three main reasons why they didn't plan to or were undecided about going back into teaching;

- 61 per cent of respondents said that it was a single factor or event that triggered their departure from the profession;

- 51 per cent of teachers who leave teaching remain in the sector.

(DfE, 2018d)

CASE STUDY

Sofia is a technology teacher and is in her sixth year of teaching. Sofia joined her current school three months ago as a head of department. Prior to this, she worked as a teacher of technology in a nearby school for five years. Within two weeks of starting her new post, the senior leadership team asked Sofia to undertake two additional responsibilities to cover a long-term staff absence. Sofia reluctantly accepted as she was keen to ensure that senior leaders saw her as ambitious and hard-working. Sofia's additional responsibilities soon began to overwhelm her and she felt that she did not have the capacity to fulfil the roles. She chose not to discuss her concerns with senior leaders as she was worried about what senior leaders would think. Eventually, Sofia began to miss deadlines and she was becoming increasingly stressed. This impacted detrimentally on her mental health, the quality of relationships and her teaching. Senior leaders began to voice their concerns about Sofia regularly missing deadlines and in response Sofia became confrontational and defensive. Sofia's relationship with senior leaders continued to break down as she had not been honest and pro-active in addressing her concerns. Equally, senior leaders had failed to recognise and identify the cause of Sofia's stress, which meant that appropriate and effective safeguards were not in place to prevent the breakdown in their relationship.

CRITICAL QUESTIONS

+ What are the attributes of an effective senior leader?
+ What might be the signs that you are being bullied or harassed by another colleague?
+ What are the attributes of an effective colleague?

MANAGING RELATIONSHIPS WITH GOVERNORS

The governors ultimately employ you to work in a school. They form the top layer of the school leadership team and they hold the headteacher to account. It is useful to know who the governors are. Governors are assigned specific areas of responsibility and you may discover that a governor has a responsibility for monitoring a specific area that you lead on. For example, you might be leading pastoral support for students and a governor may be assigned to oversee this area of school provision. If you find yourself in this situation, it is important to meet with the governor regularly and at least once each term. This will give you an opportunity to share what you are doing in relation to the role and your plans for the next term. You should be able to talk to them about what is going well and what the challenges are that associate with the role. Most governors will appreciate the opportunity to meet with you and you should not see this as a form of inspection.

Recent research by the Education Support Partnership surveyed education professionals who had experienced behavioural, physical and psychological symptoms that were due to work or where work was a contributing factor. The research was published in the Teacher Wellbeing Index (ESP, 2018) and the research demonstrated that:

- 20 per cent of those surveyed cited bullying by colleagues as a work issue that symptoms were related to;

- 28 per cent of those surveyed cited a lack of trust from managers as a work issue that symptoms were related to;

- 14 per cent of those surveyed cited a lack of opportunity to work independently as a work issue that symptoms were related to.

(ESP, 2018)

Research demonstrates that multiple factors impact on teacher well-being, including school climate (Gray et al, 2017). A negative school climate can lead to high rates of teacher absenteeism and staff turnover (Grayson and Alvarez, 2008). Evidence also suggests that there is an association between school climate and teacher and student well-being (Gray et al, 2017). Additionally, research also indicates that a positive school climate increases student academic achievement (MacNeil et al, 2009). It is possible that this is because a positive school climate results in better teacher engagement, higher levels of commitment and increased staff and student self-esteem and well-being (Gray et al, 2017). Research even suggests that a positive school climate can mitigate the negative effects of socio-economic context on students' academic success (Thapa et al, 2013). It would therefore appear that a negative school climate detrimentally impacts on the well-being of both teachers and students and has a negative impact on student attainment. Positive teacher–student relationships support students to be mentally healthy (Kidger et al, 2012; Plenty et al, 2014). These relationships help students to feel more connected to their school (Harding et al, 2019) and improve student well-being (Aldridge and McChesney, 2018) through fostering a sense of belonging. Research demonstrates that teachers with poor mental health may find it more difficult to develop and model positive relationships with their students (Jennings and Greenberg, 2009; Kidger et al, 2010). In addition, higher rates of teacher absence can impact on the quality of teacher–student relationships (Jamal et al, 2013). This is because relationships are fostered through human connection.

SUMMARY

This chapter has explored the role of school-based mentors in supporting and assessing trainees, and it has emphasised the importance of the trainee and mentor developing an effective relationship. Strategies to support the development of effective relationships have been provided. Additionally, the chapter has provided practical advice on managing relationships with colleagues, senior leaders and governors, and some critical questions have been asked in order to encourage you to reflect on your own professional relationships.

CHECKLIST

This chapter has addressed:

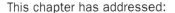

- the importance of developing effective relationships with colleagues, senior leaders and governors;
- ways of overcoming a range of common problems that you may encounter in relation to professional relationships.

FURTHER READING

Campbell, J and van-Nieuwerburgh, C (2017) *The Leader's Guide to Coaching in Schools: Creating Conditions for Effective Learning.* London: Sage.

Vass, A (2016) *Coaching in Schools Pocketbook.* Alresford: Management Pocketbooks.

✚ CHAPTER 7

MANAGING JOB APPLICATIONS AND INTERVIEWS

PROFESSIONAL LINKS

This chapter addresses the following:

🔗 TES Jobs (2007) Guides to Applying for Your First Teaching Job. TES Jobs, 8 March. [online] Available at: www.tes.com/articles/guide-applying-your-first-teaching-job (accessed 23 September 2019).

🔗 TES Jobs (2019) Why Am I Not Being Shortlisted for the Teaching Jobs I Apply For? TES Jobs, 16 September. [online] Available at: www.tes.com/jobs/careers-advice/latest-advice/teaching-job-shortlist (accessed 23 September 2019).

CHAPTER OBJECTIVES

By the end of this chapter you will understand:

+ the factors to consider when searching for and applying for teaching posts;

+ how to prepare your application and for interview;

+ how to manage stress and anxiety arising from the recruitment process;

+ how to manage disappointment and maintain resilience.

INTRODUCTION

This chapter outlines the factors that you should consider when searching for and applying for teaching posts, and it highlights the range of forums that may be used to advertise vacant positions. The chapter also emphasises the value of visiting a school to enable you to make an informed decision about whether to apply, and examples of what to look for during your visit have been highlighted for your consideration. Practical advice is offered to support your application and interview preparation, and strategies are discussed to support you to manage any stress and anxiety which you may experience throughout the recruitment process. Additionally, the chapter acknowledges that for many of us disappointment is a perfectly normal part of the application and interview process. Some advice is given to enable you to manage this, should you experience it, in order to support and maintain your resilience.

SEARCHING FOR JOBS

It can be both stressful and exciting searching for teaching posts. Posts are advertised on a range of forums, including local authority websites, the *TES* and on school websites. After narrowing down your search by phase of education (primary or secondary), you will need to consider the type of school you want to work in and the location and size of the school. Factors such as religious affiliation and whether the school is under or free from local authority control may also play a part in your decision-making process.

The person specification for the role will indicate the knowledge, skills and attributes that employers are looking for in candidates. It is worth checking these to make sure that you can meet all the minimum criteria for the post before you spend time visiting the school and applying for the job. Occasionally, people are successful in applying for jobs when they do not meet all the criteria but this is a decision that only you can make. You are more likely to be successful if you can meet all the minimum criteria and it will be an added bonus if you can meet all the desired criteria.

Before you apply for a job, it is good practice to visit the school to meet the headteacher or a senior representative. Sometimes timescales do not permit you to do this before you fill in the application but in this case you should still try to visit the school prior to the interview.

VISITING A SCHOOL

The purpose of arranging a pre-visit to the school is to enable you to make an informed decision about whether the school is right for you at this time. The visit should provide you with a reasonably clear sense of whether you will be happy working in the school. Sense the school culture to ascertain if it is a positive, happy and supportive place to work. During this visit some questions that you might consider are shown below.

+ Do the staff look happy and are they positive?
+ Do the students look happy and engaged with the school's ethos and culture?
+ Is there a positive and exciting vibe?
+ What is student behaviour like in classrooms and other spaces?
+ What is student behaviour like during social time?
+ Do you feel a sense of belonging?

If anything, the visit should calm your nerves before the interview because it will give you a good feel for the school and it will give you a chance to meet key staff. Use the visit to find out precisely what the school leaders are looking for in their preferred candidate. Also use it as an opportunity for you to decide if the school is a good fit for you.

It is a good idea to do your research prior to the visit. Take a look at the school website to see the types of activities that the school is engaging in. Download school policies and read them. Locate a copy of the recent school inspection report and from this identify the strengths of the school and its areas for development. Try not to ask questions to which the answers are already in the public domain but use your research as a springboard for finding out more during your visit, for example: *'I noticed on your website that you are doing X. Can you tell me a little more about this please?'*

Dress professionally and arrive on time. You will be more confident if you prepare a few questions to ask in advance but don't overload your host with questions. Be a good listener and do not try to play 'power games' with other candidates if they are also visiting at the same time.

APPLYING FOR JOBS

When applying for jobs, it is important to follow the instructions for completing the application exactly as stated. Do not include a curriculum vitae unless you are specifically asked for one. Pay great attention to the accuracy of your spelling, grammar, punctuation and sentence structure. Normally, applications include a two to three-page personal statement. Use this as an opportunity to address the criteria for the post by explaining how you meet these.

Tailor the personal statement to the school. Essentially, you need to communicate why you want to work in that school. Headteachers become irritated when they read standard letters of application which could be used to apply for any job. Try to link every paragraph to the school. Communicate clearly what excites you about working there and why you think you will fit into their team. You should clearly explain the knowledge, skills and other attributes that you possess and can bring to their school.

If you have completed a pre-visit, you can make reference to this in your personal statement by explaining how the visit affirmed your passion to work in the school. Also, in the personal statement, demonstrate that you have done your research by highlighting things from the school website or the Ofsted report. You will maximise your chances of success by tailoring the letter to the school while still addressing the criteria for the post. Check your paragraph structure carefully and get someone to proofread it for you before you submit it.

CRITICAL QUESTIONS

+ Should the latest school inspection grade influence whether to apply for a job in a school? Explain your answer.

+ What factors are important to you when ascertaining whether or not to apply for a job in a specific school?

THE INTERVIEW PROCESS

Most people get nervous in interviews or even at the thought of going for an interview. It is important to recognise that this is a normal reaction. When people experience a stressful situation – including a job interview – stress hormones (ie adrenaline) are triggered. In turn, this causes physiological changes in our body, including a pounding heart, rapid breathing and the appearance of sweat beads. This group of reactions is commonly referred to as our *fight-or-flight* response, which is a survival mechanism allowing us to react quickly to life-threatening and dangerous situations. The triggering of stress hormones and these physiological changes help mammals, and therefore people, to either fight a threat or flee to safety.

However, commonly, our bodies overreact to stressful experiences – including job interviews – which are in fact not life-threatening or dangerous. When you are being interviewed, you should seek assurance from knowing that your nerves are simply your body's reaction to helping you to be the best you can be. It can be helpful to try and take a positive view of this stress to reduce feelings of anxiety or panic.

During these periods of stress, it is therefore important to remember that short-term stress can benefit you during your interview.

+ Rapid breathing increases the flow of oxygen to the brain, which sharpens your senses and makes you more alert.

+ Stress releases growth hormones that increase your physical capacity to cope with demanding situations, thus increasing productivity and performance.

It is helpful to remember that our *fight-or-flight* response is automatic, but that there are a number of steps that can be taken to prepare yourself for stressful situations – including interviews. One way to keep calm in an interview is to prepare thoroughly beforehand. Use the job description and person specification to predict the questions that you might be asked. You may find it helpful to discuss your interview with friends or colleagues who have been through a similar experience or who have held, or currently hold, a similar role to the one you are applying for. Use their advice and guidance to write some bullet points down to help you to plan how you might structure your responses to any questions you are asked. There are certain standard topics that are usually addressed in interviews for teaching posts. These include safeguarding, assessment, behaviour and professional development needs. There are also many online forums that education professionals use to discuss and exchange ideas about interview preparation, including questions and suggested responses, and it is often valuable to consider browsing these websites. Other ways of trying to stay relaxed before an interview include:

+ drinking plenty of water to stay hydrated;

+ avoiding alcohol, especially the night before an interview;

+ getting plenty of sleep;

+ waking up early to give yourself plenty of time;

+ exercise;

+ eating breakfast.

CRITICAL QUESTIONS

+ Which questions would make you feel uncomfortable in an interview?

+ How can you use the support of friends, family and colleagues to help you prepare for your interview?

+ How can you change your thinking to take a positive view of stress and harness its potential power?

+ Which key topics or priorities are you likely to be questioned on in your interview?

Research by Brooks (2014) found that people who felt excited by stress-inducing social situations, for example interviews and public speaking, performed better than those who tried to remain calm throughout. The study highlights that the stress response is designed to help those experiencing stressful situations and that it can be used to our advantage. The study emphasises that it is important to recognise that nervousness and anxiety are normal feelings that are part of our *fight-or-flight* response. The research recommends taking a positive view of your stress and to see an interview as both a challenge and opportunity. It argues that those who seek to embrace this challenge and opportunity will improve their overall performance.

MANAGING STRESS AND ANXIETY DURING INTERVIEWS

As previously stated, it is normal to feel stressed and anxious during interviews, and a certain amount of stress and anxiety is necessary to help you to perform well. The problem occurs when stress and anxiety become so overwhelming that it starts to have a detrimental impact on your performance at interview.

There are strategies that you can employ to minimise stress and anxiety. These include:

+ preparing thoroughly for the interview by doing your research about the school;

+ anticipating specific interview questions;

+ thinking through possible responses to interview questions and writing these down;

+ identifying one or two questions that you might ask the panel at the end of the interview;

+ getting a good night's sleep, the night before the interview;

+ doing something relaxing before you leave the house on the day of the interview – breathing exercises, exercise, listening to your favourite music, drinking plenty of water, eating breakfast etc;

+ imagining the worst-case scenario (not getting the job) and then telling yourself that this is not the end of the world;

+ identifying the aspects of the interview that you think you will do well in and the aspects that you might struggle in (interview tasks, presentation, teaching activity, individual interview) and then preparing for these aspects thoroughly;

+ in cases of extreme anxiety, consider visiting your doctor and seeking advice.

MANAGING DISAPPOINTMENT

Naturally, you will be disappointed if you do not get the job. Your disappointment will be heightened if this is your dream job. However, it is not the end of the world and it is not life-threatening. Most people view rejection as a personal thing. However, just because you didn't get the job does not mean that you have failed. There are often many reasons why someone is rejected, and it is not always related to skill or ability level. There will be other school leaders who want to work with you and there will be other opportunities just around the corner. Sometimes it is true that things happen for a reason. It is not untypical to be unsuccessful in an interview only to secure a better opportunity quite quickly after this. Listen to the feedback, learn from it and move forward.

CRITICAL QUESTIONS

+ How do you usually manage disappointment?

+ When you have been unsuccessful in job interviews, what were the factors that contributed to this?

POSSIBLE JOB INTERVIEW QUESTIONS

General questions for teaching posts might include the following.

+ Why do you want to work in this school?

+ What skills can you bring to the job? How do you see yourself fitting in?

+ What is your approach to managing students' behaviour?

+ What would you do if you suspected that or a student disclosed that they were being abused?

+ Can you give an example of something that you have done in school that you are proud of?

+ Describe your best/worst lesson.

+ How do you use assessment to support students' progress?

Questions for middle or senior leaders might include the following.

+ Give an example of how you have made a positive impact at whole-school level?

+ What would your priorities be in the first 12 months of being appointed if you are successful?

+ How would you deal with resistance from colleagues?

+ What do you think will be the most challenging aspects of this role and how will you address the challenges?

+ What is your vision?

+ What changes would you make immediately if you are successfully appointed to this role?

+ What has been your biggest disappointment in your career? What did you learn from this?

+ What actions might you take to challenge, develop and empower those in your team or area?

- Full-time teachers are less likely to leave the system than part-time teachers, but more likely to move schools.

- Holding a more senior post in a school is associated with higher in-system retention.

- Approximately 20,000 teachers return to teaching each year, with around 60 per cent having permanent contracts compared to around 95 per cent of the remaining workforce. Returners are also less likely to work full-time.

- Most secondary teachers classed as inactive who return do so within the first few years of leaving.

- Teacher recruitment and retention statistics in England demonstrate a gender gap (24 per cent of males and 31 per cent of females return within 5 years).

- The likelihood of returning reduces with each passing year.

- The five-year retention rate of female NQTs was five percentage points higher than for male NQTs. It was also higher among those under 30.

(House of Commons, 2019)

CASE STUDY

Sarah had applied for a middle leadership post in a secondary school. She had been successfully shortlisted for the post and invited to attend an interview. The post was her dream job. It would involve managing a large science department and a significant budget. Sarah had always been ambitious. She saw this job as a stepping stone to a senior leadership position and she wanted to impress the interview panel.

Sarah was worried that she would underperform during the interview. In previous interviews, her nerves had got the better of her and this had impacted detrimentally on her progress. She had been unsuccessful in three previous interviews due to visible signs of anxiety during interviews even though she had no doubts that she would be successful in the role if she was appointed. She did not want to lose this job for the same reason. Sarah had sought feedback on her previous performances at interview and had been informed that she needed to present herself more confidently.

Sarah decided to manage her anxiety pro-actively this time. She considered the worst-case scenario, which was not getting the job. She then reflected on the implications of this; although it would certainly be disappointing, it was not life-threatening. She already had a good job that she enjoyed, she was happy in her current school and she had a reasonable salary. Getting the job would be a bonus, but it would not be the end of the world if she didn't get it.

Sarah had prepared well for the interview by identifying possible questions and she had considered possible responses to these. She had undertaken a pre-visit to the school, and this had gone well. She told herself that her appointment to the post would be a bonus not only to herself but to the school and that the school would be extremely lucky to recruit someone of her calibre. Sarah saw the interview as an opportunity for her to select the school rather than as an opportunity for the school to select her. She had read the latest inspection report and had identified ways in which she could support the school to move forward.

The night before the interview was an opportunity for Sarah to relax. She listened to her favourite music, ate a nice meal and went to bed early. She woke up early the next morning and completed some breathing activities to help her relax. She drank plenty of water to stay hydrated and blocked out negative thoughts from her mind.

The interview was successful and Sarah was offered the post.

CASE STUDY

Ryan was an NQT and he was in the process of applying for his first teaching post. He had applied for a teaching post in a school that was not far from his home, but he did not have time to arrange a pre-visit. Despite this, his application was successful, and he had been invited for an interview.

Ryan was nervous about the interview but his approach to interview preparation did not alleviate his anxiety. He did not think through the possible interview questions before the interview, he had not looked at the school website and he had not read the latest Ofsted report. His only reason for wanting to work in the school was because it was within walking distance of his home.

The night before the interview, Ryan stayed up late. He woke up late, but he still had time to attend the interview. He grabbed some clothes and got dressed but he did not have time to have a shower or eat breakfast. He forgot to take his identification to the school. By the time he got to the school he was nervous but also extremely tired.

His teaching activity had not been prepared thoroughly and did not go well. He struggled in the interview to answer the questions and many of his answers lacked depth and elicited one-word responses. He had not fully considered the reasons why he wanted to work in the school, and he could not answer this first question, which did not go down well with the interview panel. Unsurprisingly, this catalogue of errors led to Ryan not being offered the post.

- As of November 2017, the total full-time equivalent (FTE) number of teachers in publicly funded schools in England was 452,000.

- The increase in the number of teachers since 2010 has not kept pace with the increase in student numbers.

- Student numbers are projected to rise by 5 per cent between 2018 and 2024. This is driven by secondary school student numbers, which are expected to increase by 15 per cent between 2018 and 2024.

- 22 per cent of newly qualified entrants to the sector in 2015 were not recorded as working in the state sector two years later.

- In March 2016, there were around 251,000 qualified teachers aged under 60 who had previously worked in state schools in England but were no longer doing so.

(House of Commons, 2019)

Research by Frauendorfer and Schmid-Mast (2015) emphasises that there is a positive relationship between positive non-verbal behaviours and the evaluation of that candidate by the interviewer or interviewers. In the study, the researchers defined positive non-verbal behaviour as actions which elicit proximity and liking. These include, for example, a high level of eye contact, smiling, nodding and hand gestures. The researchers also highlight the role of non-verbal behaviours in creating first impressions and therefore argue that applicants can convey a first impression by expressing non-verbal behaviours during their interview. Applicants preparing for interviews may find it useful to consider the implications of the research study and reflect on any non-verbal behaviours they may be expressing.

SUMMARY

This chapter has explored the factors that you should consider when searching for and applying for teaching posts and it has highlighted the range of forums that may be used to advertise vacant positions. The chapter also emphasised the value of visiting a school to enable you to make an informed decision about whether to apply, and examples of what to look for during your visit have been highlighted for your consideration. Practical advice has been offered to support your application and interview preparation, and strategies have been discussed to support you to manage any stress and anxiety which you may experience throughout the recruitment process. Additionally, the chapter acknowledged that for many of us disappointment is a perfectly normal part of the application and interview process. Some advice is given to enable you to manage these feelings, should you experience them, in order to support and maintain your resilience.

CHECKLIST

This chapter has addressed:

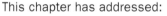 the factors to consider when searching and applying for teaching posts;

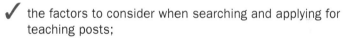 how to prepare your application and for interview;

✓ how to manage stress and anxiety arising from the recruitment process;

✓ how to manage disappointment and maintain resilience.

FURTHER READING

Alred, D (2016) *The Pressure Principle: Handle Stress, Harness Energy, and Perform When It Counts*. London: Penguin.

Hodgson, S (2015) *Brilliant Answers to Tough Interview Questions* (Brilliant Business). Harlow: Pearson.

✚ CHAPTER 8

MANAGING YOUR TIME AND WORK–LIFE BALANCE

PROFESSIONAL LINKS

This chapter addresses the following:

Department for Education (DfE) (2018) *Ways to Reduce Workload in Your School(s): Tips and Case Studies from School Leaders, Teachers and Sector Experts*. London: DfE.

CHAPTER OBJECTIVES

By the end of this chapter you will understand:

+ some practical strategies to support you in managing your time and work–life balance;

+ some of the challenges you may experience in relation to managing your workload at home and managing your personal relationships and friendships;

+ the importance of social connectivity and physical activity.

INTRODUCTION

This chapter outlines some of the common challenges that you may experience as a teacher in relation to managing your time in school effectively. The chapter argues that it is important to create opportunities for socialisation with colleagues but that it is also important to consider your time and use it productively. Additionally, it provides some practical strategies to support you in managing your time and work–life balance. The chapter also considers some of the challenges that you may experience in relation to your workload at home and in managing your personal relationships and friendships. Once again, practical advice is offered to support you in managing these demands successfully and effectively.

MANAGING TIME IN SCHOOL EFFECTIVELY

The more work that you do in school, the less work that you will have to do at home. Managing your time in school effectively will support you to achieve a good work–life balance. Schools are social places and it is important to socialise with colleagues by engaging in both work and non-work-related discussions. This is important for your well-being. However, it is also important to protect your time at school so that you can maximise your productivity.

To manage your time in school effectively, it is a good idea to think through your day. Although the majority of the day will be spent teaching students, you will have some non-contact time during the week when you can complete your wider professional duties. This will provide you with a valuable opportunity to complete administration tasks, planning, marking and other work-related duties. You will not be able to complete all your teaching-related tasks in school but it is important to effectively utilise the time that you do have. Sometimes colleagues will need to talk to you during your non-contact time and this is important. However, there will be times when you need to protect this time for your own work and you should not feel guilty about this. Although it can be difficult to follow this advice, try to put yourself first. If you spend your time supporting colleagues during the school day rather than concentrating on your own work, you will pay the price for this later because you will have to take the work home. Plan carefully how you intend to use your non-contact time each week so that this does not become time that is wasted.

Some teachers like to arrive in school early before other people arrive. This can provide a valuable opportunity to complete work when it is relatively quiet. Some teachers like to stay behind after school to complete work. It is never usually a good idea to arrive early and stay late on a regular basis because this can lead to exhaustion.

Do not feel guilty about leaving school to go home at the end of the working day. If you feel that you will be more productive working at home rather than staying behind in school then this is a sensible decision to make. You should try to allocate at least one day each week when you do leave school at a reasonable time or one morning each week when you arrive later than usual. Ultimately, decisions about how best to use your time in school are personal and you will find a way of working that suits you.

If you are a senior or middle leader you will have a significant workload. You may spend some time teaching, a lot of time in meetings and time carrying out monitoring activities. You may need to spend significant amounts of time supporting your colleagues. However, you should protect some time each day when you can complete your own work and you should not feel guilty about this. Some leaders like to operate 'open-door' policies so that colleagues and students can access them. However, this limits opportunities for meeting your own workload commitments so it might be better to use 'office hours' in which you make yourself available to others at specific times. There may be times when you simply need to close the office door and get on with your work, especially when you have important deadlines to meet. It is perfectly reasonable to support staff during the working day and to allocate some protected time after school to address your own workload. Again, if you spend all of your time supporting colleagues, you will pay the price by taking work home with you.

You should not be afraid to say to colleagues that you are unable to support them immediately but you will be able to meet them at a specific time. No-one will protect your time for you. You have to do it yourself. Other people will happily fill your diary with meetings, but ultimately you will need to decide whether to accept or reject the meeting, depending on your own work-related commitments. Sometimes you will have no choice, and you will have to attend meetings and meet with colleagues and these activities will take you away from your own workload. However, sometimes it is perfectly acceptable to say 'no' to people and people should respect your right to do this.

MANAGING WORKLOAD AT HOME

Teaching will inevitably require you to complete work at home. There are simply not enough hours in the day to complete all of your work in school and you will find that you need to work in the evenings, at weekends and during holidays to keep on top of your job.

Although most teachers generally accept that they will need to work at home, it is important to decide how much of your own time you are prepared to spend on work. Some teachers arrive home, start working immediately and finish work in the evening. Others work all through the evening and into the night. Sometimes you may need to do both! Many teachers have family responsibilities which restrict the amount of work that they can do at home. Teachers who have parenting responsibilities may be forced to complete work-related tasks after their children have gone to bed.

The point is that the amount of work you do at home is dependent on your personal circumstances at the time. Life gets in the way sometimes and you have to accept this. It is important to draw some boundaries by deciding how much time you are prepared to spend on work-related tasks at home. It is acceptable for you to restrict the number of hours you are prepared to spend on work at home. It is perfectly reasonable to identify days of the week when you will not do any work at home and it is absolutely essential that you make time to do activities unrelated to work. You should not feel that you need to spend all of your weekend working. Some teachers allocate a day at the weekend when they do not do any work. There may be weekends when you have to work on both days and you should certainly have some free weekends when you do not do any work. Your line manager cannot direct the amount of time you spend on work outside of school. You will need to make an informed professional decision about how much time to allocate to your work and you should never feel guilty for not working in your free time.

CRITICAL QUESTIONS

+ What are the advantages and disadvantages of undertaking work-related tasks at home?

+ How can you use your working day more productively to minimise the amount of work that you need to take home?

CASE STUDY

Rhonda is a full-time middle leader and has two young children. Prior to having children, Rhonda would regularly stay late at school to prepare resources and work through her to-do list. Rhonda knew that as a parent she would need to leave work much earlier and she believes that self-discipline is key. Rhonda follows a tight schedule for the activities she completes during planning, preparation and assessment (PPA) time and this allows her to leave school on time for four evenings per week. Rhonda stays late once per week, as her wife takes their children to a local swimming class. Once a month, Rhonda rotates her schedule so that she can watch her children at their swimming class. Rhonda believes that it is crucial to be organised and disciplined and she feels that having a rigid schedule is crucial to her work–life balance.

MANAGING YOUR PERSONAL RELATIONSHIPS AND FRIENDSHIPS

Spending time with partners, friends and family is important for your well-being. Being a teacher is only part of your identity, although some teachers do make it their whole identity. Spending time with others on non-work-related activities is important for your well-being and therefore it is important to protect time for this. Relationships with others are important, particularly when teachers are experiencing stress in the workplace. Family, friends and partners can be a source of support in these situations, particularly if teachers feel that they are unable to talk to colleagues at work.

However, personal relationships do not necessarily have a positive effect on well-being. Glazzard and Rose (2019) interviewed teachers who had experienced difficulties in personal relationships as a result of domestic violence and sustaining these relationships had a detrimental impact on their well-being. In addition, they found that when family members became ill or required additional care this had a detrimental impact on the well-being of teachers and resulted in them not being able to meet their professional commitments to the standard that they were used to. Some of these teachers felt torn between their jobs and their personal commitments, particularly when family members became ill. They experienced exhaustion and eventually burnout after trying to fulfil their personal and professional obligations (Glazzard and Rose, 2019).

THE IMPORTANCE OF SOCIAL CONNECTIVITY AND PHYSICAL ACTIVITY

The World Health Organization (2014) defines mental health as:

…a state of well-being in which every individual realizes his or her own potential, can cope with the normal stresses of life, can work productively and fruitfully, and is able to make a contribution to her or his community. Health is a state of complete physical, mental and social well-being and not merely the absence of disease or infirmity.

Physical and social well-being therefore form part of one's overall well-being. Glazzard and Rose (2019) found that teachers in their study participated in physical activity and invested time in social networks as key coping strategies to mitigate the effects of work-related stress.

You may feel that sometimes you need to neglect these activities in order to meet your professional commitments but neglecting physical activity and opportunities to socialise with others can be detrimental to your overall health. It is not wise to neglect these for long periods of time. Try to build small amounts of physical activity into each day. A short, brisk walk every day for 20 minutes can be extremely beneficial because over the duration of a week this totals 140 minutes of moderate to vigorous activity. Regular participation in physical activity will increase your energy levels, reduce exhaustion and help you to feel more alert in the classroom. Maintaining a healthy diet will also help you to keep physically fit. Examples of strategies for staying physically healthy include:

+ walking or cycling to school;

+ joining the school sports club;

+ using the stairs in school rather than the lift;

+ participating in the 'daily mile' with students;

+ walking the dog;

+ walking to the shops rather than driving.

The physical and mental health benefits of engaging in physical activity for adults as well as children and young people are well documented and widely and internationally accepted (Ahmed et al, 2016; Hyndman et al, 2017; McMahon et al, 2017; Yun Wu et al, 2017). Physical activity can enhance social and emotional functioning and health-related quality of life, and develop protective factors including self-esteem, positive social relationships and well-being (Fraser-Thomas and Côté, 2009; Holt, 2016).

CRITICAL QUESTIONS

+ What types of physical activity do you participate in?

+ What are the barriers to participating in social networks and physical activity?

+ How can these barriers be overcome?

According to the Teacher Wellbeing Index (ESP, 2018):

● teacher work–life balance was affected by working long hours on weekdays (stated by 71 per cent of teachers), not finding time to be with family/friends (65 per cent), working over the weekends (62 per cent) and working during the holidays (60 per cent);

● conversely, 26 per cent stated that family commitments were a factor in preventing them doing a good job at work.

CASE STUDY

Dianne is a primary school teacher and is in her ninth year of teaching. In her first years of teaching, Dianne found it difficult to maintain a work–life balance and would often decline invitations to social events so that she could continue to work through her ongoing to-do list. Dianne realised in her sixth year of teaching that her work–life balance was unsustainable, and she shared these concerns with a trusted colleague. Her colleague encouraged her to recognise and accept that her to-do list would never be fully achieved and that there would always be work tasks to complete. Dianne now considers tasks in terms of urgency and importance, and plans dedicated time for personal commitments rather than working through tasks continuously one after another. She feels that she has found a new balance and that her new lifestyle makes her professional work more rewarding.

According to research:

Many of the teachers interviewed talked about wanting to be perfect or in control. One even confessed to being borderline OCD (obsessive compulsive disorder). It would appear there is a certain characteristic trait in some teachers that drives them to deliver everything to perfection and to maintain control; at times when this is not possible they become anxious and stressed.

(Glazzard and Rose, 2019, p 23)

Prioritisation and organisation appear to be key skills that those [teachers] prone to poor mental health often reported learning after they had had a crisis; a sign that beforehand they were seeking perfection and thought they could (and should) do everything all of the time. They came to realise that this is not always possible and sometimes there have to be compromises.

(Glazzard and Rose, 2019, p 30)

According to the Teacher Wellbeing Index (ESP, 2018):

- 74 per cent of education professionals consider the inability to switch off and relax to be the major contributing factor to a negative work–life balance;

- more than half (58 per cent) of all education professionals work more than 41 hours per week;

- senior leaders work much longer hours than they are contracted to do – only 5 per cent are contracted to work 51+ hours per week and yet 59 per cent do so;

- teachers work longer hours than they are contracted to do as well – only 6 per cent are contracted to work 41–50 hours per week but 25 per cent do, and only 2 per cent are contracted to work 51+ hours per week and yet 29 per cent do;

- working long hours and the feeling of stress appear to be closely linked. The highest levels of stress reported come from those professionals working more than 41 hours per week, whereas those working less than 40 hours per week were more likely to report not feeling stressed.

SUMMARY

This chapter has explored some of the common challenges that you may experience as a teacher in relation to managing your time in school effectively. The chapter has argued that it is important to create opportunities for socialisation with colleagues but that it is also important to consider your time and plan your productivity. Additionally, it has provided some practical strategies to support you in managing your time and work–life balance. The chapter then considered some of the challenges that you may experience in relation to your workload at home and in managing your personal relationships and friendships. Once again, practical advice has been offered to support you in managing these demands successfully and effectively.

CHECKLIST

This chapter has addressed:

✓ some practical strategies to support you in managing your time and work–life balance;

✓ some of the challenges you may experience in relation to managing your workload at home and managing your personal relationships and friendships;

✓ the importance of social connectivity and physical activity.

FURTHER READING

Holmes, E (2018) *A Practical Guide to Teacher Wellbeing*. London: Sage.

Mann, A (2018) *Live Well, Teach Well: A Practical Approach to Wellbeing That Works*. London: Bloomsbury.

✛ CONCLUSION

This book has attempted to provide you with practical solutions to help you manage your workload and time, develop your resilience, establish strong relationships and achieve a better work–life balance.

It is refreshing that the issue of teacher workload is high on the political agenda. Steps are currently being taken to reduce workload in Initial Teacher Training ITT and for qualified teachers working in schools. It is also reassuring that the government has created a special advisory group to specifically look at teacher well-being. At the same time, the Ofsted framework for schools has been revised so that inspectors give greater emphasis to how school leaders are addressing the issue of teacher workload.

At the same time, there is also a new focus in school inspections which gives inspectors the power to investigate issues of staff bullying. We have argued in this book that the issue of teacher workload only provides a partial perspective on the factors which contribute to poor teacher mental health. Teachers thrive when they work within positive school cultures where they are trusted, valued and assigned agency. We have argued that toxic school cultures can have a detrimental impact on the mental health of teachers and also on students. Although it is admirable that inspectors will be assigned power to investigate this issue, we are concerned that teachers who work within toxic environments may not feel that they can talk to inspectors about their negative experiences. How likely is it that a teacher will disclose to an inspector that that they are being bullied by another colleague or a senior leader if this jeopardises the outcome of the inspection and ultimately their career? Although promises of anonymity may be made, these may not be sufficiently reassuring to the individual who has to continue to work in the school following the inspection.

Issues of teacher stress are influenced by a combination of factors, including negative and toxic school climates. These climates are shaped by school leaders who themselves are influenced by a challenging educational policy climate. Senior leaders also experience significant stress due to the performative-driven educational discourse in which they operate. Sometimes, they transmit this stress on to teachers and teachers then transmit it on to students. Therefore, the problem of teacher well-being requires a systemic approach which critically examines and deconstructs the factors in the wider education system which contribute to poor teacher mental health.

Teachers thrive (and work hard) when they are respected, trusted and valued. Ethical and moral leadership embraces these principles. It is unlikely that there will be an imminent change to the wider education policy climate which detrimentally impacts on teacher mental health. However, school leaders do have the power to shape school cultures and to buffer some of the stress which teachers are exposed to. They make a decision about the type of leader they are going to be and how to treat people who work within their schools. Although individual teachers can take practical steps to enable them to be mentally healthy, the school climate ultimately influences their day-to-day experiences within the school. We therefore argue that the issues of poor teacher mental health extend beyond workload and that there should be a greater focus on establishing a mentally healthy school culture for senior school leaders.

✚ REFERENCES

Ahmed, M D, King, W, Ho, Y, Zazed, K, Van Niekerk, R and Jong-Young Lee, L (2016)
The Adolescent Age Transition and the Impact of Physical Activity on Perceptions of Success, Self-Esteem and Well-Being. *Journal of Physical Education and Sport*, 16(3): 776–84.

Aldridge, J M and McChesney, K (2018)
The Relationships Between School Climate and Adolescent Mental Health and Wellbeing: A Systematic Literature Review. *International Journal of Educational Research*, 88: 121–45.

Beck, A, Crain, A L, Solberg, L I, Unützer, J, Glasgow, R E, Maciosek, M V and Whitebird, R (2011)
Severity of Depression and Magnitude of Productivity Loss. *Annals of Family Medicine*, 9(4): 305–11.

Beltman, S, Mansfield, C and Price, A (2011)
Thriving Not Just Surviving: A Review of Research on Teacher Resilience. *Educational Research Review*, 6(3): 185–207.

Bethune, A (2018)
Wellbeing in the Primary Classroom. London: Bloomsbury Education.

Brooks, A W (2014)
Get Excited: Reappraising Pre-Performance Anxiety as Excitement. *Journal of Experimental Psychology: General*, 143(3): 1144–58.

Brunetti, G J (2006)
Resilience Under Fire: Perspectives on the Work of Experienced, Inner City High School Teachers in the United States. *Teaching and Teacher Education*, 22(7): 812–25.

Day, C (2008)
Committed for Life? Variations in Teachers' Work, Lives and Effectiveness. *Journal of Educational Change*, 9(3): 243–60.

Day, C and Gu, Q (2007)
Variations in the Conditions for Teachers' Professional Learning and Development: Sustaining Commitment and Effectiveness over a Career. *Oxford Review of Education*, 33(4): 423–43.

Department for Education (DfE) (2011)
Teachers' Standards Guidance for School Leaders, School Staff and Governing Bodies. London: DfE.

Department for Education (DfE) (2016a)
Reducing Teacher Workload: Marking Policy Review Group Report. London: DfE.

Department for Education (DfE) (2016b)
Reducing Teacher Workload: Data Management Review Group Report. London: DfE.

Department for Education (DfE) (2017a)
Teacher Workload Survey 2016. London: DfE.

Department for Education (DfE) (2017b)
Case Studies of Behaviour Management Practices in Schools Rated Outstanding. London: DfE.

Department for Education (DfE) (2018a)
School Workforce in England: November 2017. London: DfE.

Department for Education (DfE) (2018b)
Addressing Teacher Workload in Initial Teacher Education (ITE): Advice for ITE Providers. London: DfE.

Department for Education (DfE) (2018c)
Permanent and Fixed Period Exclusions in England: 2016 to 2017. London: DfE.

Department for Education (DfE) (2018d)
Factors Affecting Teacher Retention: Qualitative Investigation. London: DfE.

Department for Education (DfE) (2018e)
Ways to Reduce Workload in Your School(s): Tips and Case Studies from School Leaders, Teachers and Sector Experts. London: DfE.

Department for Education (DfE) (2019)
Early Career Framework. London: DfE.

Dodge, R, Daly, A, Huyton, J and Sanders, L (2012)
The Challenge of Defining Wellbeing. *International Journal of Wellbeing*, 2(3): 222–35.

Doney, P A (2012)
Fostering Resilience: A Necessary Skill for Teacher Retention. *Journal of Science Teacher Education*, 24(4): 645–64.

Education Support Partnership (ESP) (2018)
Teacher Wellbeing Index 2018. London: ESP.

Fraser-Thomas, J and Côté, J (2009)
Understanding Adolescents' Positive and Negative Developmental Experiences in Sport. *The Sport Psychologist*, 23(1): 3–23.

Frauendorfer, D and Schmid-Mast, M (2015)
The Impact of Nonverbal Behaviour in the Job Interview. In Kostić, A and Chadee, D (eds) *The Social Psychology of Nonverbal Communication* (pp 220–47). Basingstoke: Palgrave Macmillan.

Glazzard, J and Coverdale, L (2018)
It Feels Like It's Sink or Swim: Newly Qualified Teachers' Experiences of Their Induction Year. *International Journal of Learning, Teaching and Educational Research*, 17(11): 89–101.

Glazzard, J and Rose, A (2019)
The Impact of Teacher Wellbeing and Mental Health on Pupil Progress in Primary Schools. Leeds: Leeds Beckett University.

Gray, C, Wilcox, G and Nordstokke, D (2017)
Teacher Mental Health, School Climate, Inclusive Education and Student Learning: A Review. *Canadian Psychology*, 58(3): 203–10.

Grayson, J L and Alvarez, H K (2008)
School Climate Factors Relating to Teacher Burnout: A Mediator Model. *Teaching and Teacher Education*, 24(5): 1349–63.

Greenfield, B (2015)
How Can Teacher Resilience Be Protected and Promoted? *Educational and Child Psychology*, 32(4): 52–69.

Griffiths, S (2011)

Being Dyslexic Doesn't Make Me Less of a Teacher. School Placement Experiences of Student Teachers with Dyslexia: Strengths, Challenges and a Model for Support. *Journal of Research in Special Educational Needs*, 12(2): 54–65.

Gu, Q and Day, C (2013)

Challenges to Teacher Resilience: Conditions Count. *British Educational Research Journal*, 39(1): 1–23.

Haggarty, L and Postlethwaite, K (2012)

An Exploration of Changes in Thinking in the Transition from Student Teacher to Newly Qualified Teacher. *Research Papers in Education*, 27(2): 241–62.

Harding, S, Morris, R, Gunnella, D, Ford, T, Hollingworth, W, Tilling, K, Evans, R, Bell, S, Grey, J, Brockman, R, Campbell, R, Araya, R, Murphy, S and Kidger, J (2019)

Is Teachers' Mental Health and Wellbeing Associated with Students' Mental Health and Wellbeing? *Journal of Affective Disorders*, 242: 180–7.

Harrison, J K (2001)

The Induction of Newly Qualified Teachers. *Journal of Education for Teaching*, 27(3): 277–9.

Hobson, A J, Malderez, A, Tracey, L, Homer, M, Mitchell, N, Biddulph, M, Giannakaki, M S, Rose, A, Pell, R G, Roper, T, Chambers, G N, and Tomlinson, P D (2007)

Newly Qualified Teachers' Experiences of Their First Year of Teaching: Findings from Phase III of the Becoming Teacher Project. Nottingham: University of Nottingham.

Holt, N (2016)

Positive Youth Development Through Sport (2nd ed). London: Routledge.

Hong, J Y (2012)

Why Do Some Beginning Teachers Leave the School, and Others Stay? Understanding Teacher Resilience through Psychological Lenses. *Teachers and Teaching*, 18(4): 417–40.

House of Commons (2019)

Teacher Recruitment and Retention in England. London: House of Commons.

122

Huisman, S, Singer, N R and Catapano, S (2010)
Resiliency to Success: Supporting Novice Urban Teachers. *Teacher Development*, 14(4): 483–99.

Hyndman, B, Benson, A C, Lester, L and Telford, A (2017)
Is There a Relationship Between Primary School Children's Enjoyment of Recess Physical Activities and Health-Related Quality of Life? A Cross-Sectional Exploratory Study. *Health Promotion Journal of Australia*, 28: 37–43.

Jain, G, Roy, A, Harikrishnan, V, Yu, S, Dabbous, O and Lawrence, C (2013)
Patient-Reported Depression Severity Measured by the PHQ-9 and Impact on Work Productivity: Results from a Survey of Full-Time Employees in the United States. *Journal of Occupational and Environmental Medicine*, 55(3): 252–8.

Jamal, F, Fletcher, A, Harden, A, Wells, H, Thomas, J and Bonell, C (2013)
The School Environment and Student Health: A Systematic Review and Meta-Ethnography of Qualitative Research. *BMC Public Health*, 13(1): 798.

Jennings, P A and Greenberg, M T (2009)
The Prosocial Classroom: Teacher Social and Emotional Competence in Relation to Student and Classroom Outcomes. *Review of Educational Research*, 79(1): 491–525.

Kidger, J, Araya, R, Donovan, J and Gunnell, D (2012)
The Effect of the School Environment on the Emotional Health of Adolescents: A Systematic Review. *Pediatrics*, 129(5): 2011–48.

Kidger, J, Brockman, R, Tilling, K, Campbell, R, Ford, T, Araya, R, et al (2016)
Teachers' Wellbeing and Depressive Symptoms, and Associated Risk Factors: A Large Cross Sectional Study in English Secondary Schools. *Journal of Affective Disorders*, 192: 76–82.

Kidger, J, Gunnell, D, Biddle, L, Campbell, R and Donovan, J (2010)
Part and parcel of teaching? Secondary school staff's views on supporting student emotional health and well-being. *British Educational Research Journal*, 36(6): 919–935.

Kyriacou, C (2001)

Teacher Stress: Directions for Future Research. *Educational Review*, 53(1): 27–35.

Le Cornu, R (2009)

Building Resilience in Preservice Teachers. *Teaching and Teacher Education*, 25(5): 717–23.

Le Cornu, R (2013)

Building Early Career Teacher Resilience: The Role of Relationships. *The Australian Journal of Teacher Education*, 38(4): 1–16.

MacNeil, A J, Prater, D L and Busch, S (2009)

The Effects of School Culture and Climate on Student Achievement. *International Journal of Leadership in Education*, 12(1): 73–84.

McMahon, E, Corcoran, P and O'Regan, G, et al (2017)

Physical Activity in European Adolescents and Associations with Anxiety, Depression and Well-Being. *European Child and Adolescent Psychiatry*, 26(1): 111–22.

National Education Union (NEU) (2017)

Workload Survey. London: NEU.

National Education Union (NEU) (2018)

Teachers and Workload. London: NEU.

National Foundation for Educational Research (NFER) (2016)

NFER Teacher Voice Omnibus. London: NFER.

Office for Standards in Education (Ofsted) (2019)

The Education Inspection Framework. Manchester: Ofsted.

Papatraianou, L H and Le Cornu, R (2014)

Problematising the Role of Personal and Professional Relationships in Early Career Teacher Resilience. *Australian Journal of Teacher Education*, 39(1): 100–16.

Plenty, S, Östberg, V, Almquist, Y B, Augustine, L and Modin, B (2014)

Psychosocial Working Conditions: An Analysis of Emotional Symptoms and Conduct Problems Amongst Adolescent Students. *Journal of Adolescence*, 37(4): 407–17.

Schonfeld, I S (2001)

Stress in 1st-Year Women Teachers: The Context of Social Support and Coping. *Genetic, Social, and General Psychology Monographs*, 127(2): 133–68.

Sfard, A and Prusak, A (2005)

Telling Identities: In Search of an Analytic Tool for Investigating Learning as a Culturally Shaped Activity. *Educational Researcher*, 34(4): 14–22.

Skaalvik, E M and Skaalvik, S (2009)

Does School Context Matter? Relations with Teacher Burnout and Job Satisfaction. *Teaching and Teacher Education*, 25(3): 518–24.

Skinner, B F (1938)

The Behavior of Organisms: An Experimental Analysis. New York: Appleton-Century.

Stansfeld, S A, Rasul, F, Head, J and Singleton, N (2011)

Occupation and Mental Health in a National UK Survey. *Social Psychiatry and Psychiatric Epidemiology*, 46(2): 101–10.

Tait, M (2008)

Resilience as a Contributor to Novice Teacher Success, Commitment, and Retention. *Teacher Education Quarterly*, 35(4): 57–75.

TES (2007)

Guides to Applying for Your First Teaching Job. TES Jobs, 8 March. [online] Available at: www.tes.com/articles/guideapplying-your-first-teaching-job (accessed 23 September 2019).

TES (2019)

Why Am I Not Being Shortlisted for the Teaching Jobs. TES Jobs, 16 September. [online] Available at: www.tes.com/jobs/careers-advice/latest-advice/teaching-jobshortlist (accessed 23 September 2019).

Thapa, A, Cohen, D, Guffey, S and Higgins-D'Alessandro, A (2013)

A Review of School Climate Research. *Review of Educational Research*, 83(3): 357–85.

Totterdell, M, Woodroffe, L, Bubb, S, Daly, C, Smart, T and Arrowsmith, J (2005)

What Are the Effects of the Roles of Mentors or Inductors Using Induction Programmes for Newly Qualified Teachers (NQTs) on Their Professional Practice, with Special Reference to Teacher Performance, Professional Learning and Retention Rates? In *Research Evidence in Education Library* (1–77). London: EPPI-Centre, Social Science Research Unit, Institute of Education.

Totterdell, M., Woodroffe, L, Bubb, S and Hanrahan, K (2004)

The Impact of NQT Induction Programmes on the Enhancement of Teacher Expertise, Professional Development, Job Satisfaction or Retention Rates: A Systematic Review of Research on Induction. In *Research Evidence in Education Library* (1–59). London: EPPI-Centre, Social Science Research Unit, Institute of Education.

University of Nottingham (2011)

Beyond Survival: Teachers and Resilience. Nottingham: University of Nottingham.

Wilson, D (2004)

The Interface of School Climate and School Connectedness and Relationships with Aggression and Victimization. *The Journal of School Health*, 74(7): 293–9.

World Health Organization (WHO) (2014)

Mental Health: A State of Well-Being. [online] Available at: www.who.int/features/factfiles/mental_health/en/ (accessed 11 August 2019).

Yun Wu, X, Hui Han, L, Zhang, J H, Luo, S, Hu, J W and Sun, K (2017)

The Influence of Physical Activity, Sedentary Behaviour on Health-Related Quality of Life Among the General Population of Children and Adolescents: A Systematic Review. *PLOS ONE*, 12(11): 1–29.

+ INDEX